Pha

Calculations Made Easy

PTCB & NAPLEX Test and Exam Prep for Pharmacy Technicians

PLUS 2 FULL Practice Tests

Richard Douglas

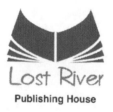

Lost River
Publishing House

COVER DESIGN

ERICA ANDERSON

FIRST EDITION

Contents

Calculations in Pharmacy

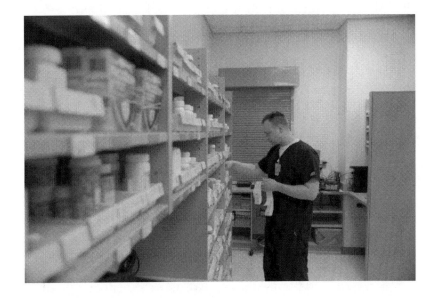

Accurate calculations in pharmacy can prevent medical errors; further underdosing may lead to subtherapeutic treatment, and overdosing may lead to drug toxicity. In addition, calculations in pharmacy also require knowledge of commonly used units. For example, certain medications are dispersed in ml or mg, whereas others are dispensed in volumes (ml). Vitamins, for example, are available in international units.

Drugs are administered via various routes that include oral, IM, IV, SC, topical, etc. The route of administration must be considered when making dose calculations to ensure safety. For example, the oral dose of a drug is usually much higher than the same drug given intravenously; Thus, if your IV dose is larger than the oral dose, you need to recheck your calculations.

Further pharmacy calculations are also of importance for outpatients. Patients need to be educated about the differences between a tablespoon and a teaspoon and how much volume they contain. Further, the patient must be taught what one ml is.

In order to correctly administer therapeutic doses of medications to patients, calculations are vital in pharmacy. Both the pharmacist and pharmacy technician who dispense medications need to know the exact concentration of drugs that are being given to patients. In addition, they need to know how to calculate correct doses and prepare and compound medications accurately.

Definitions

In order to understand calculations in pharmacy, it is important to understand the below definitions:

Dose: This refers to the medication dose which is supposed to be consumed at a set time

Dosage: Refers to the administration of a drug, the amount, frequency and number of doses that are consumed over a defined time

Concentration: Refers to the amount of active ingredients per total weight of a drug

Alligation: Is a process that involves mixing solids or solutions of different strengths. The technique is used to derive another solution or solid with the same active ingredient in both but of a different strength.

Specific gravity: This refers to the ratio of substance weight compared to the weight of an equal volume of water. For example, specific gravity is measured as the number of grams of a substance/number of milliliters of a substance. by knowing the specific gravity, the weight or volume can then be determined.

Tonicity: Refers to how an extracellular solution can alter the cell volume by affecting osmosis. The tonicity of a solution correlates directly with the osmolarity of the solution. Osmolarity, in turn, refers to the total concentration of the solute in the solution.

Apothecary: Is an old system of measurements first used in Greece. It has now been replaced by the metric system, including the dram and grain.

Body surface area (BSA): Refers to the total body surface area, taking into account the individual's height and weight and expressed in m2

% Strength: Reflects the number of grams contained in 100 ml of solution. It is very useful to know. For example, a 1% lidocaine solution contains 1 gram of lidocaine in 100 ml of water/saline.

% Weight in Volume: Is expressed as percentage w/v. It is actually the number of grams in 100 mL solution. Substances or powdered drugs are suspended in a liquid and then calculated as w/v.

% Volume in Volume Expressed as percentage v/v: this refers to the amount of milliliters added to a 100 mL of solution.

% Weight in weight: When two semi-solids or powders are mixed, this is expressed as percentage w/w. It refers to the number of grams in 100 grams of solution. Ointments are usually calculated in this manner.

Dilutions: The relationship between volume and concentration is inversely proportional. For example, if a solution needs to be diluted, the active drug concentration in the solution does not change, but the volume will increase.

Isotonicity: When two solutions have equal salt concentration, and osmotic pressure is said to be isotonic. Normal saline is an isotonic crystalloid solution with a concentration of 0.9% (w/v) of sodium chloride in sterile water.

Essential Symbols

% percent; usually part per hundred

+ plus or add; or positive

- minus or subtract; or negative

/ divided by

x multiple or times

< value on the right is bigger than the value on the left or the left value is smaller than the right value (e.g., 4 < 5)

> value on the right is smaller than the value on the left or the left value is bigger than the right value (e.g., 5 > 4)

= is equal to; equals

. decimal point

, decimal marker (comma)

a:b ratio symbol (e.g., a:b)

How to Use SI Units Correctly

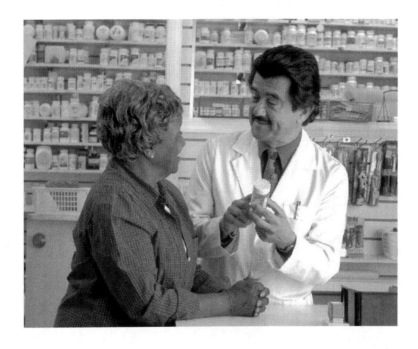

1. Symbols and unit names should not be capitalized except when used as a heading or at the beginning of a sentence. The exception is the symbol L for liter, which may or may not be capitalized. For example, 3 L or 3 l, 3 g and 3 mm-not 3G and 3Mm.

2. In North America, the decimal point (.) is usually placed in between the denomination and denominate number (e.g., 3.5 mL). But in some European countries, a

comma or a raised dot may be used. (eg 3,5 mL or 3·5 mL)

3. Unless you are at the end of a sentence, periods are not used following SI symbols. Example 3 mL and 3 mg, NOT 3 mL. or 4 mg.

4. If you have a compound unit that is a quotient or a ratio of 2 units, this should be indicated by a solidus (/) or a negative exponent. For example, 4 ml/h and not 5 ml per hour.

5. If you use a symbol in one expression, then the symbols should be continued. For example, if you write 2 mg/ml, you should not write 2 mg/milliliter.

6. Use of plurals. For example, you can write 3 milliliters or 3 ml but not 3 mls. When you write symbols for SI units, the letter denotes both plural and singular values. There is no need to place an 's' when their value or item is bigger or more. For example, 1mg or 10 mg.

7. You can write micrograms in two ways: mcg or µg.

8. To prevent drug errors, one should place a zero in front of the leading decimal point. This can hopefully prevent drug errors caused by uncertain decimal points. For

example, 03 mg and not .3 mg. Pharmacy professionals must be able to recognize a misplaced or misread decimal point as it can lead to an error in calculation or dispensing ten times the quantity. For example, 1.0 can be interpreted as 10. To avoid medication errors, a trailing zero should not follow a whole number. For example, 4 mg and not 4.0 mg.

9. In general, when writing dimensions, be concise. For example, instead of writing 400 g, you may want to write 0.4 kg, or instead of 800 ml, write 0.8 L.

Use of Abbreviations and Symbols

1. Abbreviations have been used in pharmacies for ages and are still visible on medication orders and prescriptions.

2. While some abbreviations have been derived from Latin, many others have evolved from healthcare workers who wanted to create shortcuts.

3. Medication errors related to abbreviations are very common.

4. The general rule is that abbreviations should be avoided. Write the text in full.

Recommendations for Reducing Medication Errors

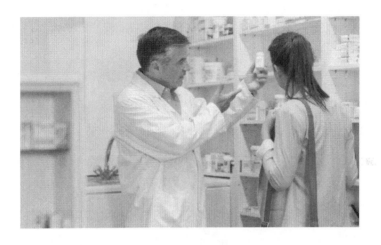

1. When writing a whole number, do not use a decimal point or a terminal zero. For example, 9 milligrams should be written as 9 mg and not 9.0 mg.

2. If the unit or quantity is smaller than one, it should have a zero preceding the decimal point. For example, three-tenths of a gram should be written as 0.3 g and not as .3 g.

3. A single space should always be left between the number and the unit. For example, 50 g and not 50g.

4. Try to use whole numbers whenever possible and avoid using equivalent decimal fractions. For example, 200 mg and not 0.2 g.

5. Always use the full names of medications. For example, do not write Dig; instead, spell it out like digoxin.

6. Establish a trend for using USP designations for all units of measure. For example, when stating milligrams, use mg and not mgm or mgs.

7. Spell out the word units in full. For example, do not write regular insulin 5 U. Instead, write regular insulin 5 units. The letter U can be misread.

8. Do not use the abbreviation IU for international units. It can easily be mistaken or misread for IV or intravenous.

9. Abbreviations for the eyes and ears should never be used. Instead, spell out the right eye instead of using the abbreviation o.d.

10. Never use abbreviations like 'q.d' for every day; it can be misread as q.o.d or q.i.d, which can lead to a major medication error.

11. Avoid using the abbreviation 'd' for a day; it can be mistaken for dose.

12. Boost the healthcare provider's direction on the prescription label when necessary and for clarity. For example, instead of just saying 'one tablet in a.m,' write it out - 'swallow one tablet in the morning with water.'

13. Finally, keep up to date with guidelines and recommendations from the Institute for Safe Medication Practices (ISMP). The agency regularly publishes a list of symbols and abbreviations that it recommends for discontinuation.

Decimals

Besides fractions, the use of decimals in pharmacy is common. Decimals generally represent quantities less than one or quantities between two whole numbers. For example, 0.5 of an item means one-half of the item. All numbers to the left of the decimal point represent whole numbers, and numbers to the right of the decimal point represent quantities less than one.

When decimals are not used correctly, they can result in medication errors. In addition, stray pen marks, sloppy writing, and poor-quality faxed or scanned copies can also lead to misinterpretation. To avoid medication errors, pharmacy professionals should follow a standard approach when using decimals.

1. Only use decimals if absolutely necessary. For example, ten milligrams should be written as 10 mg and not 10.0 mg. The use of a decimal point and trailing zero are not necessary.

2. Secondly, only zeros that serve as placeholders should be included after the decimal. For example, if you want to write two and four hundredths, you should write it as 2.05

with no zeros following the last significant digit.

3. Thirdly, a decimal point should not be written without a number before it. For example, if you want to write half a gram, it should be written as 0.5g, and not .5g. Failure to use a leading zero can lead to an error in the interpretation of the dose- .5 g could be interpreted as 5 g.

The bottom line is that use a ZERO always to lead but never to trail.

Decimals are also widely used in pharmacy; they are usually converted into fractions. Thus the technician should become familiar with basic arithmetics that includes ratios, fractions, proportions, and percentages.

Fractions

Pharmacy professionals must know how to convert fractions to decimals. While this can be done with a calculator, it is important to know how to perform the task manually. For example, if you have a fraction of ⅔, you can convert it to a decimal by dividing two by 3. The decimal is 0.666. Another example of a fraction converted to a decimal is 1 ¼ is written as 1.25.

In the majority of pharmacy calculations, decimals are usually rounded to the tenth or hundredth, depending on the scenario. To round a number to the

In most pharmacy calculations, decimals are rounded to tenths (most common), hundredths, or thousandths, depending on the situation. To round to the tenth, look at the number in the tenth place; if it is 5 or larger, then you can round off the adjacent number to 1. For example, if you have the number 1.26, 6 is greater than 5, so you can round off the 2 to a 3, giving 1.3.

On the other hand, if you have the number 1.23, then 3 is less than 5, and the number can be written as 1.2.

Rounding off is necessary because some numbers are not practical or measurable. For example, you will never encounter a dose of 2.5112 mL of a medication.

In most cases, the milliliter (mL) number is rounded to the close ml of a tenth of an ml. For example, if the calculation reveals 1.67mL, this can be rounded off to 1.7 ml.

Common fractions that are often converted to decimals include:

1/4 = 0.25

1/2 = 0.5

3/4 = 0.75

1/5 = 0.2

2/5 = 0.4

6/8 = 0.75

4/5 = 0.8

Percentages

Percentages are a composite of decimals and fractions. The percentage usually means 'per 100.' Fractions are usually changed into a percentage by multiplying by 100, or the percentage can be changed into a decimal by moving the point.

For example, 91% = 0.91.

To convert a decimal into a percentage, simply multiply by 100. For example, 0.25 = 0.25 x 100 = 25%

Density

- Defined as mass per unit volume of a substance.

- Density is usually expressed as grams per cubic centimeter (g/cc).

- Because the gram is defined as the mass of 1 ml of water at 4 C, the density of water is 1 g/ml.

- In contrast, one milliliter of mercury weighs 13.6 g; hence, its density is 13.6 g/mL.

Density can be calculated by dividing mass by volume, that is:

- Density = Mass/Volume

Q. If 20 ml of hydrochloric acid weighs 32 g, the density is:

- Mass (32 g)/volume (20 ml) = 1.6 grams per milliliter

Specific Gravity

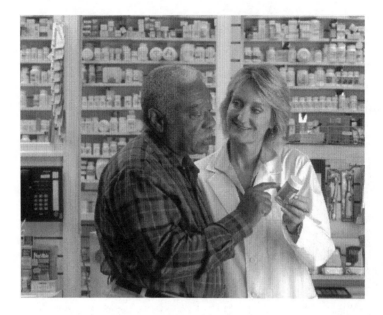

1. Specific gravity (sp gr) is a ratio that is expressed decimally of the weight of a substance to the weight of an equal volume of a substance chosen as a standard, both substances at the same temperature.

2. Water is used as the standard for the specific gravities of liquids and solids; the most helpful standard for gases is hydrogen.

3. Specific gravity may be calculated by dividing the weight of a given substance by the weight of an equal volume of water, that is:

Specific gravity is the Weight of substance/weight of an equal volume of water

1. Substances with a specific gravity of less than 1 are lighter than water.

2. Substances that have a specific gravity greater than 1 are heavier than water.

Calculating Specific Gravity of Liquids

To calculate the specific gravity of a liquid when its volume and weight are known involves the use of the equation:

Specific gravity = Weight of substance/Weight of equal volume of water

Q. If 45 ml of oil weighs 44 g, what is the specific gravity of the oil?

• Weight of substance (44 g)/weight of an equal volume of water (45 ml) = 44/45

• Hence: Specific gravity = 0.977

Q. What is the weight in grams of 200 ml hydrochloric acid, with a specific gravity of 1.18 g/ml?

• 200 ml of water weighs 200 ml. therefore, 200 x 1.18 = 236 g

In addition, the volume can also be calculated by knowing the specific gravity and weight.

Q. What is the volume in milliliters of 492 g of hydrochloric acid with a specific gravity of 1.18?

• The formula is sp gr = weight of substance/weight of an equal volume of water

• 1.18 = 492/X

• Therefore x = 416 ml

Q. What is the volume in milliliters of 1 pound of salicylic acid with a specific gravity of 1.35?

• A pound equals 454 g

• Therefore 1.35 = 454/X

• X = 336 ml

Q. What is the cost of 1,000 mL of hydrogen peroxide, specific gravity 1.01, bought at $45 per pound?

- Sp gravity = weight/weight of an equal amount of water

- $1.01 = x/1,000$ ml

- x =1,010 g

- The cost is $45 for 1 pound or 454 g

- Therefore 1,010 g will cost $1,010/454 \times \$45 = \$100.10$

Ratios and Proportions

Ratios reveal the relationship between the items. Ratios are commonly used in pharmacies. For example, many drugs are based on the patient's body weight. The dose is usually written as mg/kg or milligrams per kilogram. Frequently two ratios with similar units are combined to create proportions or otherwise known as a statement of equality between the two ratios.

When attempting to solve proportions, it is important to make sure that the equation is set up correctly before you solve for the unknown variable.

For example, the standard dose of an antibiotic is 5 mg per kg. If a patient weighs 100 kg, what will be the total dose for the patient?

- 5 mg/kg = 100 times x

- Therefore x = 5 x 100= 500 mg

Q. A solution of an antibiotic has 10 mg in 5 ml. How many mg will be present in 10 ml of the solution?

- Set up a proportion and solve for x:

- 10 mg/5 ml= x mg /10

- x = 20mg

Examples of Weight-in-Volume Calculations

Q. How many grams of dextrose will be required to prepare 2000 ml of 7.5% solution?

- 7.5% means that there is 7.5 g per 100 ml

- Hence in 2,000 ml, there will be 2,000/100 x 7.5 = 150 g of dextrose

Q. How many grams of potassium chloride will be used in compounding the following prescription? Potassium chloride 0.2% in 250 ml of sterile water?

- 0.2% means that there is 200 mg in every 100 ml.

- To make 250 ml, 250/100 x 200 mg = 500 mg or 0.5 kg

W/V Calculations

Q. What is the percentage strength (w/v) of solution X if

70 ml contains 10 g?

- 70 ml of water weighs 70 g

- Hence 70/10 =100/X

- Therefore x = 14.2%

Q. How many milliliters of a 4% solution can be made from 30 g of sodium bicarbonate?

- 4% is equal to 4 g

- Therefore, 30/4 = x/100 x = 750 g.

- If the solution is in water, this is 750 ml

Percentage Volume-in-Volume

Liquids are usually measured by volume, and the percentage strength indicates the number of parts by volume of an ingredient contained in the total volume of the solution or liquid preparation considered as 100 parts by volume. If there is any possibility of misinterpretation, this kind of percentage should be specified: e.g., 10% v/v.

Example of v/v Calculations

Q. How many milliliters of liquefied sodium hydroxide should be used in compounding the following prescription?

- Liquefied sodium hydroxide 5%

- Urea lotion add 240 mL

Volume (mL) % (expressed as a decimal) milliliters of active ingredient

- 240 mL/100 = x/5 =x = 12 mL.

Q. An elixir contains 10% v/v of honey. What volume of the elixir will contain 50 ml of alcohol?

- 10 (%)/100 (5%) = 50 (ml)/x

- x = 500 ml

Percentage Weight-in-Weight

Percentage weight-in-weight (true percentage or percentage by weight) indicates the number of parts by weight of active ingredient contained in the total weight of the solution or mixture considered 100 parts by weight.

Examples of w/w Calculations

Q. How many grams of urea should be used to prepare a 120 g of a 5% (w/w) solution in water?

• Weight of solution (g) 120

• 5% expressed as a decimal = 0.05

• Thus, 120 x 0.05 = 6 g

Measurement Systems

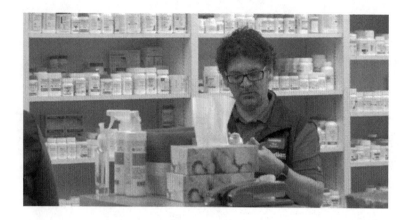

There are several systems of measurement in pharmacy, but the most common is the metric system, also referred to as the international system of units (SI). All pharmacy professionals need to know how to convert the metric system into avoirdupois, apothecary, and other household systems.

Metric System (International System of Units)

The metric system is globally utilized and is the accepted system of measurement in most pharmacies. The system is based on multiples of ten. The standard units used in healthcare are:

- gram (mass: microgram, milligram, or gram)

- meter (distance: millimeter, centimeter, or meter)

- liter (volume: ml, liter)

The key relationship among these units is that 1 mL of water occupies one cubic centimeter and weighs 1 gram.

Prefixes are also used to indicate the unit's relationship to the standard unit. For example, milli stands for one thousandth, or one milliliter is 1/1,000 of a liter.

Solid medications are usually stated in grams or milligrams. Liquid medications are stated as mL or liters. If the volume or dose of a medication is not commercially available, the right amount needs to be compounded- but doing so needs knowledge about conversions between the units of the metric system.

When medication orders are filled, the technician must pay attention to the units to prevent errors and harm to the patient.

When using the metric system, movement of the decimal to the right or left of the number will present as a decrease or an increase in the size of the unit. Once you know the order of prefixes and the size each represents, one can easily convert from one metric unit to another.

For example:

- 0.005 kg = 5 grams = 5,000 mg = 5,000,000 micrograms

Example: Ciprofloxacin 400 mg tablet

- 1 tablet = 0.4 g = 400mg = 40,000 mcg

The pharmacy professional should know the different types of metric units like ounces, pounds, and kilos, as frequent conversions are necessary since many drug doses are based on body weight.

Common conversions used in pharmacy include:

- 1 kg = 2.2 pounds

- 30 g = one solid ounce

- 15 ml = 1 tablespoon

- 5 ml = 1 teaspoon

- 30 ml = 1 liquid ounce

- 1 gram = 1,000 mg

- 1 mg = 1,000 micrograms

Conversions are also required for temperature and time. For example, to convert degree Celsius to Fahrenheit, you divide by 5, then multiply by 9 and add 32.

To convert Fahrenheit to Celsius, you first subtract 32, multiply by 5 and then divide by 9.

Ratio Strength

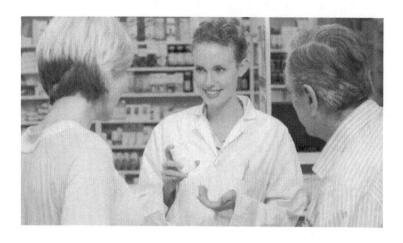

The concentrations of weak solutions are frequently expressed in terms of ratio strength. Because all percentages are a ratio of parts per hundred, ratio strength is another way of expressing the percentage strength of solutions or liquid preparations (and, less frequently, of mixtures of solids). For example, 5% means five parts per 100 or 5 g. Although five parts per 100 designate a ratio strength, it is customary to translate this designation into a ratio, the first figure of which is 1; thus, 5:100 or 1:20.

When a ratio strength, for example, 1:1,000, is used to designate a concentration, it is to be interpreted as follows:

• For solids in liquids, 1 g of solute or constituent in 1,000 mL of solution or liquid preparation.

• For liquids in liquids, 1 mL of the constituent in 1,000 mL of solution or liquid preparation.

• For solids in solids, 1 g of the constituent in 1,000 g of mixture.

The ratio and percentage strengths of any solution or mixture of solids are proportional, and either is easily converted to the other by proportion.

Ratio strength and percentages are also frequently used in pharmacy calculations.

To calculate most doses, the pharmacist will need to know the following:

• Size of the dose

• Number of doses

• Frequency of administration

In most cases of calculation, the same equation can be

used, but the terms may need to be rearranged depending on what is being asked. No matter what equation you use, the units of volume or weight have to be the same for the size and total quantity of the dose.

Q. How many grams of sodium chloride are needed to make 500 ml of a 1:100 solution?

• First, convert 1:100 into a percentage which is 1%

• This means that every 100 ml contains 1 g, and thus, 500 ml will require 5 g of sodium chloride

Q. If the dose of a drug is 100 mg, how many doses are contained in 2 g?

• First, convert 2 g into milligrams; = 2000 mg

• If each dose is 100 mg, then you will need to divide 2000 mg by 100= 20 doses

Q. A patient is prescribed two tablespoonfuls of a liquid medication twice a day for five days. How many milliliters in total will you dispense?

• Number of doses = 10 (twice a day for five days)

- The size of the dose is two tablespoonfuls or 30 ml (each tablespoonful is 15 ml)

- Total quantity is 10 x 30 ml = 300 ml

Q. The pharmacist has asked you to prepare 50 dosage forms of a drug, each containing 15 mg. What is the total number of milligrams you will need?

- Number of doses required = 50

- The size of each dose is 15 mg

- Total = 50 X 15 = 750 mg

Roman Numerals

Because Roman numerals are difficult to alter, they are still widely written on prescriptions; All pharmacy technicians should be able to recognize the first 100 roman numerals.

Common roman numerals that the pharmacy technician should know include the following

l 1

ll 2

lll 3

lV 4

V 5

Vl 6

Vll 7

Vlll 8

lX 9

X 10

After 10, the roman numerals are followed by

Xl 11

Xll 12

Xlll 13, etc

XX 20

In addition, there are also other roman numerals that have higher integer values like

L 50

C 100

D 500

M 1,000

Aliquot Method

When one wants to dilute a drug with a solution or mix two different concentrations of solutions, the aliquot method is widely used. In general, an aliquot is a method to distinguish a large sample and break it into many smaller parts. In addition, aliquoting is also sensitive to temperature changes.

Stock Solutions

Stock solutions are often used to prepare or break up large amounts of drugs into small amounts before they can be dispensed to the patients. Stock solutions exist because some patients do require different concentrations of drugs.

The alligation method helps the technician calculate and dispense the correct concentration of an active ingredient to the patient.

For example:

Q. If 0.030 g of a chemical is used to prepare 100 tablets, how many micrograms will be contained in each tablet?

- First, convert 0.03 g into milligrams which is 30 mg, and then convert this to micrograms which is 30,000 micrograms.

- The total number of tablets is 100; hence a single tablet will contain

30,000 mcg/100 = 300 micrograms

Q. A cough mixture contains 3 g of a drug in 100 ml. How many grams are contained in each tablespoonful dose?

- 1 tablespoonful = 15 ml

- 1 ml will contain 3 g (3,000 mg) / 100 ml = 30 mg

- Hence 30 mg x 15 ml = 0.45 g

Q. How many grams of an antibiotic are needed to make 150 ml of a solution if each teaspoon contains 2 mg of the substance?

- Each teaspoon is 5 ml

- Hence in 150 ml, there are 30 teaspoons

- Each teaspoon contains 2 mg, and thus 30 teaspoons

will contain 60 mg

Q. A healthcare provider has ordered 250 mg capsules of an antibiotic to be taken three times a day for seven days. How many total grams of the antibiotic will be dispensed?

• The size of dose is 250 mg

• Total number of doses 3 (a day) for 7 (days) = 21 doses

• Total quantity: 250 mg x 21 (doses) = 5,250 mg or 5.25 g.

Q. The pharmacy has a stock solution of one pint (473 ml). The dose for each patient is one tablespoon. How many doses are contained in the stock?

• One pint is 473 ml

• One tablespoon is 15 ml

• Thus, the number of doses is 473/15 ml = 31 doses

Q. The pharmacy has just received a stock supply of a drug that weighs 100 g. How many doses will be available if each patient receives 0.4 g?

- 0.4 g = 400 mg

- 100 g = 100,000 mg

- Thus, 100,000/400 = 250 doses

Q. The stock contains an elixir of 200 ml contained in 20 doses. How many teaspoonfuls would be prescribed with each dose?

- The size of the dose is 200 ml

- There are 20 doses

- So each dose = 10 ml

- Each teaspoonful is 5 ml, so 10 ml would be two teaspoonfuls

Body Weight

Since the dosing of many drugs is based on body weight, it is important to understand what body surface area (BSA) is. There is a slight difference between BSA and BMI. The Body Mass Index (BMI) reflects the individual's fat mass, whereas the BSA provides the total surface area of the individual's body. The BSA is often used to calculate the drug dosage and volume of fluids that need to be administered intravenously.

There are many formulas to calculate BSA but the most widely used method is the Du Bois and Du Bois formula which states that:

Body Surface Area = 0.007184 x (Height(m)0.725) x (Weight(kg)0.425)

In some patients, the drug dosage may be based on the BSA, depending on the properties of the drug. The average BSA in an adult male is 1.7 m^2 and in a female is 1.6 m^2

BSA is calculated as follows:

- BSA (m^2) = [Height (inches) x Weight (lbs)/3131]1/2.

Calculating drug dose based on weight

1. The majority of drugs are dosed based on body weight

2. The result is expressed as mg/kg since most drugs are administered in milligram amounts

3. Always convert pounds to kilos first

Q. The initial dose of a cancer drug is 300 mcg/kg of body weight. How many milligrams will be needed to treat a 175-pound male? Hint: always check the units to ensure that you are dealing with kilograms.

Solving the equation:

- 300 mcg = 0.3 mg

- The patient's weight is 175 pounds which divided by 2.2 is 79.5 kg

- Hence the patient will need 79.5 kg x 0.3 mg =23.8 mg

Q. The average dose of a particular drug for children older than two months is between 50-75 mg/kg of body weight.

What will the dose range be for a child who weighs 50 pounds?

• First, convert pounds to kilos; hence 50 pounds is 22.7 kg

• The dose range is between 50-75 mg/kg

• Hence for 50 mg/kg, the dose =1,136 mg

• For 75 mg/kg, the dose = 1,650 mg

Hence the dose range will be between 1,136 to 1,650 mg.

Calculating Dose by Body Surface Area

The body surface area can also be used to calculate drug doses. This method is frequently used in cancer patients being administered chemotherapy and children, with the exception of neonates- who are dose based on weight and other features like biochemical, functional, physical, and pathological factors.

• It is important to know that the average BSA in an adult is 1.73m2.

Q. If the adult dose of a drug is 150 mg, calculate the approximate dose for a child with a BSA of 0.80 m2.

- 0.80/1.73 x 150= 69.3 mg

Clark and Young Rules

To calculate medication doses in children, one may use Clark's or Young's rule. Young's rule is based on patient age, whereas Clark's rule is based on the child's weight.

- Clark's rule: (Weight divided by 150 lbs.) x adult dose = Pediatric dosage.

- Young's rule: [Age / (Age + 12)] x recommended adult dose = Pediatric dose.

Factors that Influence Pharmacy Calculations

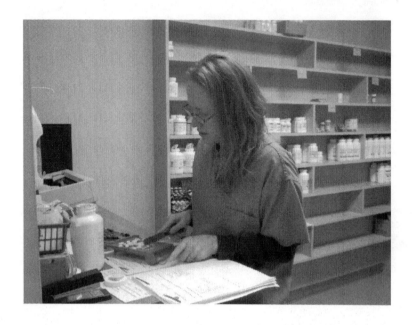

Despite ensuring correct drug dosages, one should not forget that there are other pharmacokinetic factors that may influence drug levels. For example, the bioavailability of the drug is profoundly affected after oral administration; further rates of drug excretion and metabolism can also influence drug levels in the body.

Correct and accurate pharmacy calculations are not only important for dosing, dispensing, and properly medicating patients but are also a critical component of therapeutics and patient care. Different patient populations may have varying responses to medications/ in addition, advanced age and kidney and liver dysfunction may also alter the drug metabolism. Finally, the accuracy of pharmacy calculations also are important for patient outcomes; at the same time, we have a very litigious society that is ready to sue for every little mistake or error.

Parts Per Million

When the strengths of solutions are very diluted, they are often expressed as part per million (ppm) or parts per billion (ppb); this means that there is one part per 1 million or 1 billion parts. For example, fluoride is added to the drinking water to prevent cavities, but the levels of fluoride are very low and vary from 1-6 parts per million (i.e., 1:1,000,000 to 6: 1,000,000).

In addition, metals and other chemicals that are found in small amounts in our drinking water are also expressed as parts per million. And this applies to many chemicals, pesticides, herbicides, microorganisms, etc. The levels of these agents are usually followed to ensure that they are not increasing in the environment/water supply.

In pharmacy, calculations of parts per million are often

used as either ratio strength or percentage strength.

For example, ten parts per million is the same as 1: 100,000 ratio strength and 0.0001% in percentage strength.

Q. A drug additive added to animal feed has a concentration of 15 ppm. How many milligrams of the drug are needed to prepare 5 kg of feed?

• 15 ppm is 15 g in 1,000,000 g feed.

• Thus, 15 x 5 kg (5000 g)/1,000,000 = 75 mg

Drug Doses

1. Dose: The amount of drug that is taken by the individual to derive the intended therapeutic effect. The dose is usually stated as a single treatment, the daily dose, the amount of drug that is consumed at a set time, or the total dose.

2. Daily dose: May be subdivided if taken 2-6 times a day depending on the illness and drug characteristics.

3. Drug regimen: When there is a schedule of dosing (e.g., three times a day for five days), it is referred to as a drug

regimen.

4. Quantitatively, the doses of drugs vary; some drugs have small doses and others have large doses to obtain the therapeutic effect.

5. The dose of a drug depends on its biochemical properties and pharmacological activity, its chemical and physical properties, dosage form, route of administration, and patient characteristics.

6. The dose of a drug for a specific patient is often determined based on the patient weight, age, body surface area, general health, and the presence of liver or kidney disease.

7. Drug dosing in cancer patients and some young children is highly specialized and individualized. In cancer patients, combination therapy is common, and hence the dose of each drug is adjusted according to the response. Cancer drugs are also administered in cycles of 3- 4 weeks to allow the body to recover from the adverse effects of the drugs.

8. The median effective dose is a dose of the drug that generates a specified therapeutic response in 50% of the

recipients. The ED50 is a practical method of comparing drug potencies that generate pharmacologically similar effects at different concentrations.

General Features of Dose Calculations

1. Liquid medications need to be accurately measured, and patient education is necessary since caregivers often administer drugs to children and the elderly.

2. A teaspoonful has a capacity of 5 ml.

3. A tablespoonful has a capacity of 15 ml.

4. The household teaspoons are not accurate for measuring drug volumes as the capacity for teaspoons can vary from 3 to 7 ml, and the tablespoon capacity can vary from 14-22 ml.

5. Oral dispensers for measuring liquid medication are available in most pharmacies and should be recommended to caregivers who treat children at home.

Biologicals and Units of Activity

There are dozens of pharmaceutical products made from biological sources like animals, cell cultures, plants, and biotechnology. The potency of these biological products is based on units of activity. The units of activity are set by comparing to known standard biological products. In general, there is a correlation between the unit of activity of a biological product and a measurable effect. The unit of activity may be defined as units per milliliter or units per milligram. The units of activity are often used in proportion or a ratio to determine either the volume or weight contained in a set number of units.

The following formula is often used:

Units of activity (given)/ Weight or volume (given) = Units of activity (given or desired)/ Weight or volume (given or desired)

Pharmacy-Based Immunizations and Units

Over the past decade, pharmacists in North America have been approved to administer vaccines as part of their professional activities. However, before a pharmacist or a technician can administer the injections, he or she has to undergo immunization training and be aware of the established protocols and guidelines. Calculations of biological material or its potency are usually done with the use of proportions and ratios or dimensional analysis.

For example:

Q. How many milliliters of U-100 insulin are required to obtain 30 units of insulin?

• U-100 insulin contains 100 units/mL

• 0.1 ml contains 10 units

• Hence to obtain 30 units, one needs 0.3 ml

Q. The healthcare provider has ordered 100 units of insulin to be added to 250 ml of D5W to treat a patient with diabetic ketoacidosis. How many milliliters of the insulin injection concentrate U-500 should be utilized?

• 500 insulin contains 500 units/ml

• This means there are 50 units in every 0.1 ml

- To add 100 units, one needs to aspirate 0.2 ml of the U-500 concentrate

Q. A patient with a pulmonary embolus needs to be heparinized. How many milliliters of heparin sodium injection containing 100,000 units in 20 ml should be used to obtain 10,000 units of heparin?

- Heparin 100,000 units in 20 ml

- Hence 100,000/20 = 5,000 units in each ml

- To obtain 10,000 units of heparin, aspirate 2 ml of the concentrate

Activity Based on Weight

Q. A patient requires a topical antibiotic. The physician has ordered neomycin sulfate with a potency of 500 ugs per milligram. How many milligrams of the neomycin sulfate will be equivalent to 1 mg of neomycin?

- Formula: 500 ug/1,000 ug = 1 mg/x mg

- Therefore x = 2 mg

Biological Agents Calculations

Q. An 8-year-old child has been ordered tetanus toxoid. The biological product contains 75 Lf units of tetanus toxoid in 2.5 ml. If a healthcare provider has ordered 10 Lf of toxoid for the child, how many milliliters will be administered?

Formula:

- 75 Lf units/10 Lf = 2.5 ml/x ml

- X= 0.33 ml

Heparin Dosing Calculations

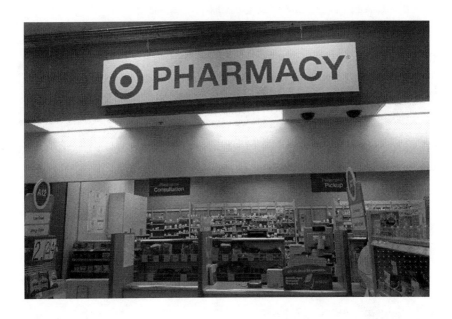

Heparin is a mucopolysaccharide with anticoagulant properties. The agent can decrease the clotting time and is often used to treat deep vein thrombosis and pulmonary embolism. Heparin sodium is standardized to contain 140 USP heparin units in each milligram. Heparin is usually administered intravenously or as a subcutaneous injection. When heparin is administered to patients in therapeutic doses, its dose is adjusted based on laboratory levels of blood coagulation parameters like partial thromboplastin time (PTT). The normal PPT varies from

32-39 seconds. Heparin has a very short half-life, and the blood levels of PTT are measured every 4-6 hours. In general, the PTT should be maintained at 1.5 to 2 times the patient's pretreatment baseline level.

Heparin is administered in several ways: IV bolus followed by an intravenous drip or subcutaneous injection. In general, heparin is widely used as a prophylactic treatment to prevent DVT after surgery. The usual dose is 5,000 units every 4-6 hours.

Much higher doses of heparin are required to treat active phlebitis, pulmonary embolism, and prevention of deep vein thrombosis after hip replacement. In children, the dose of heparin may be 50 mg/kg via intravenous drip or 20,000 units/m^2 every 24 hours. Most hospitals have protocols for heparin use, and pharmacists must follow the institution's practice guidelines.

Besides heparin, there are also several low molecular weight heparins (LMWHS) that are also used as antithrombotic agents. For example, both dalteparin sodium (Fragmin) and Enoxaparin sodium (Lovenox) are widely used both in and out of the hospital. The LMWHs are also administered subcutaneously, have a lesser tendency to affect platelet function, and tend to have a more predictable anticoagulant response. Most importantly, they do not require monitoring of clotting time.

Heparin Dosing

1. The recommended dose of the LMWH dalteparin in patients undergoing orthopedic procedures is 2,500 IU within 2 hours of surgery.

2. When heparin or LMWH are administered, all intramuscular injections must be stopped; otherwise, the patient can form a massive hematoma.

3. Patients generally do not receive aspirin when administered heparin or LMWH.

4. The pharmacist or the pharmacy technician should always check the PTT before renewing an order for heparin. The therapeutic PTT value should be between 50-70 seconds or twice the baseline level.

Examples of Heparin Dose Calculations

Q. The physician has ordered heparin at a rate of 1,000

units per hour for a 140-pound patient. The intravenous infusion contains 20,000 units of heparin sodium in 500 ml of D5W. What is the concentration of heparin sodium in units/ml?

• There are 20,000 units in 500 ml of D5W.

• Therefore, 1 ml will contain 20,000/500 = 40 units of heparin.

Q. The physician has ordered heparin at a rate of 1,000 units per hour for a 140-pound patient. The intravenous infusion contains 20,000 units of heparin sodium in 500 ml of D5W. What will be the duration of the drip?

• 20,000 units in 500 ml at a rate of 1000 units per hour.

• The duration of the drip will be 20,000 units divided by 1,000 units per hour= 20 hours.

Q: A 170-pound patient has been ordered heparin for a deep vein thrombosis in the left leg. The physician states that the patient should receive an initial heparin bolus (50 units/kg) followed by a heparin drip (10 units/kg/hr) for the first 6 hours. The total amount of heparin the patient will be administered is?

- First, convert pounds to kilos

- 170 pounds divide by 2.2 = 77 kg

- The bolus is 50 units per kg = 50 x 77 kg= 3,863 units of heparin

- Then he receives a heparin drip of 10 units/kg for 6 hours.

- This equals 10 units x 77 kg x 6 hours= 4,620 units of heparin

- Thus, the total amount of heparin he receives is 3,863 + 4,620 = 8,483 units of heparin

Renal Dysfunction and Dose Calculations

In patients with renal dysfunction, the kidneys are unable to excrete the drug. This can result in toxicity if high doses of drugs are used. In general, polar or water-soluble drugs are commonly excreted by the kidney, and their excretion is affected when the kidney is not functioning.

In general, in people with renal dysfunction, creatinine levels are carefully monitored. Higher levels of serum creatinine signal that the kidney function is declining, and hence drug dose adjustments are necessary. There are several formulas that can be used to calculate the dose of drugs in the presence of renal dysfunction, and it is important to consult with a nephrologist when this happens. In addition, all drugs that worsen renal function have to be discontinued or their doses adjusted.

Laboratory Data and Drug Calculations

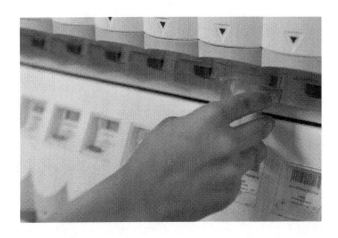

While in healthy people, there may not be a need to check the laboratory data before dispensing a drug, in most chronic patients, the laboratory data must be checked before prescribing the medication. It is now common practice to check urine, electrolytes, glucose, bilirubin, liver, and renal function before prescribing medications to chronically ill patients or those who have a chronic illness.

For example, in a patient with hypertension who is on an angiotensin-converting enzyme inhibitor, the presence of renal function can quickly lead to elevations in potassium-which in turn can lead to deadly arrhythmias. Hence either the drug dose needs to be altered or the drug discontinued, and another drug with no effect on real function started. Type 1 diabetics constantly monitor their blood sugar levels and adjust the insulin dosage depending on the levels.

Another example is in patients with hypercholesterolemia who are prescribed statin drugs. The dose of the drug usually depends on the levels of cholesterol, and the treatment is often for many months or years. But it is vital to monitor levels of serum cholesterol because the dose may have to be reduced if the levels of cholesterol drop. While statins are relatively safe drugs, they can cause life-threatening myositis and mild cases of liver dysfunction. In such scenarios, drug therapy with statins has to be discontinued.

The learning point is that in people on long-term drug therapy or those with chronic disorders, the pharmacy professional must check the laboratory values of the different parameters before dispensing the drug. Often the dose of the drug has to be adjusted or discontinued when specific laboratory abnormalities are identified.

Q. A 62-year-old diabetic male is found to have serum

cholesterol levels of 300 mg/dl. How many milligrams of cholesterol will be present in a 20 ml sample of the patient's serum?

- 300 mg/dl = 300 mg/100 ml;

- Therefore, every ml contains 3 mg

- In 20 ml, there will be 20 ml x 3 mg = 60 mg

Tonicity

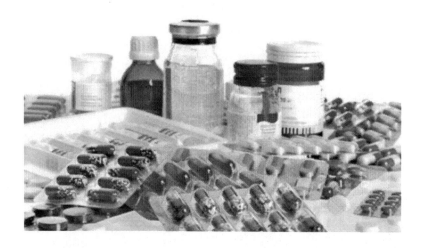

When a dilute solution passes through a semipermeable membrane into a concentrated solution, with time, the concentration of the two solutions will be equal. This biochemical phenomenon is known as osmosis.

The pressure that drives the dilute solution to move past the semipermeable membrane is termed the osmotic pressure. The osmotic pressure varies depending on the chemical nature of the solute. Non-electrolyte solutions only contain molecules, and the osmotic pressure depends on the concentration of the solute. On the other hand, solutions made of electrolytes contain ions, and the osmotic pressure depends on the concentration of the solute and the degree of dissociation. The higher the rate of dissociation, the greater the osmotic pressure.

When two solutions have similar osmotic pressure, they are known as isosmotic. The majority of solutions used for patient treatment have similar osmotic pressure to body fluids which ensures better efficacy, improved patient comfort, and safety.

When two solutions have the same osmotic pressure, they are termed isotonic (meaning equal tone). In general, pharmaceutical preparations are made isotonic to match the body fluids.

Solutions that have lower osmotic pressure than a comparable body fluid are called hypotonic, whereas those that have a higher osmotic pressure are termed hypertonic.

When preparing pharmaceutical dosages intended to be mixed with biological fluids of the nose, eye, bowel, or bladder, isotonicity has to be taken into consideration.

Why Tonicity Matters

1. In general isotonic solutions are acceptable for IV and ophthalmic administration as they are better tolerated

compared to hypertonic or hypotonic solutions.

2. For example, isotonic artificial tears are much better tolerated than hypotonic tears.

3. When isotonic fluids are administered, there is homeostasis in the intracellular fluids of the body.

4. In rare cases, hypertonic fluids may be used to draw fluids out of edematous tissues.

Tonicity and Patient Considerations

It is important to have the right tonicity, especially for parenteral and ophthalmic solutions. The reason is that isotonic solutions are better tolerated compared to hypo or hypertonic solutions. When isotonic solutions are injected, there is immediate homeostasis with the body's intracellular fluids. On the other hand, when hypo or hypertonic fluids are administered to the eye or intravenously, they can cause significant irritation, pain, and discomfort.

For the most part, isotonic fluids are preferred for administration to patients.

However, there are a few exceptions; For example, hypertonic solutions are sometimes administered to draw fluids out of the tissues.

Milliequivalents

Milliequivalents are widely used in North America to express the concentration of electrolytes in a solution. A milliequivalent is coupled to the final number of ionic charges in a solution; it also is dependent on the ionic valency. In simple terms, a milliequivalent is a unit of measurement that reflects the degree of chemical activity of an ionic substance (e.g., KCL, NaCl, etc.).

In European nations, instead of milliequivalent, the molar concentration is used.

Under normal physiological and stable body conditions, the blood plasma contains an equal number of cations (positively charged ions) and anions (negatively charged ions). The total concentration of anions always equals the total concentration of cations. For example, any number of milliequivalents of K, Na, or any cation will always react with precisely the same number of milliequivalents of HCO3, Cl, or any anion.

For any given chemical compound/solution, the milliequivalents of anions equal the milliequivalents of cations equals the milliequivalents of the chemical compound. For example, when preparing a solution of Na ions, sodium salt is dissolved in water. Besides the Na ions, there will also be ions of a negative charge in the solution, which is usually chloride. The two components of sodium chloride will be chemically equal in that the milliequivalents of sodium are equal to the milliequivalents of chloride.

The key point to understand is that when you dissolve enough sodium chloride in water to obtain 40 mEq of Na per liter, you also have exactly 40 mEq of chloride. However, in the final solution, the weight of each ion will differ.

A milliequivalent reflects the amount in milligrams of a solute that is equal to $1/1,000$ of its gram-equivalent weight; it also takes into account the ionic valence. In general, the milliequivalent expressed the combined power or chemical activity of a solution/substance relative to the activity of 1 mg of hydrogen. Therefore based on the valence and atomic weight of the substance, one mEq represents 1 mg of hydrogen, 23 mg of sodium, 20 mg of calcium, 39 mg of potassium and so on. These are standard numbers readily available on the internet.

In intravenous fluids and other solutions used in medicine, the electrolyte concentrations are usually expressed as mEq/L. To convert the concentration of electrolytes in solution expressed as milliequivalents per unit volume to weight per unit volume and vice versa, use the following:

To convert milligrams (mg) to milliequivalents (mEq):

• mEq = mg x Valence divided by Atomic formula or molecular weight

To convert milliequivalents (mEq) to milligrams (mg):

• mg = mEq x Atomic, formula, or molecular weight divided by Valence

To convert milliequivalents per milliliter (mEq/mL) to milligrams per milliliter (mg/mL):

• mg/mL = mEq/mL x Atomic, formula, or molecular weight divided by Valence

Q: A 60-year-old obese male has a serum cholesterol level of 300 mg/dl. What is the equivalent value expressed in millimoles per liter?

- First, 300 mg/dl is the same as 3,000 mg/L

- The molecular weight of cholesterol is 387 mg

- To convert mg to millimoles, use the formula:

- 3, 000 mg x 1 mEq divided by 387 = 7.76 mmol/L

Q.A 62-year-old diabetic male is found to have serum cholesterol levels of 300 mg/dl. What is the equivalent expressed in terms of milligrams percent?

- You have 300 mg/dl

- Next convert to milligram percent= 300 mg/100 x 100 = 300 mg%

Q: If a solution contains four mEq of potassium chloride per milliliter, what is the concentration in milligrams per milliliter?

- The molecular weight of KCL = 74.5

- The equivalent weight of KCL = 74.5

- Hence one mEq of KCL = 74.5 g/1,000 = 0.0745 g or 74.5 mg

• Therefore, four mEq of KCL will contain 74.5 x 4 = 298 mg/ml

Q: You are given a solution of calcium chloride that contains 2 mEq per milliliter. How do you express this in terms of grams per liter?

• The formula weight of CaCl2 = 147

• Equivalent weight of CaCl2 = 147/valence = 147/2 = 73.5

• 1 mEq of CaCl2 = 73.5/1,000 = 0.0735 g or 73.5 mg

• Therefore 2 mEq of CaCl2 contains 0.0735 x 2 = 0.147 g/ml

Q: You have been given a solution containing 100 mEq of sodium chloride. What is the percent (w/v) concentration of the solution per liter?

• The molecular weight of NaCl is 58.44

• The equivalent weight of NaCl is 58.44

• 1 mEq of NaCl = 58.44/1,000 = 0.05844 g

• 100 mEq equals 0.05844 x 100 = 5.84 g/L or 0.585 g/100 ml

Q: You have been given a solution that contains 20 mg/100 ml of Mg ions. Express this concentration in terms of milliequivalents per liter.

• The atomic weight of Magnesium is 24

• The equivalent weight of Magnesium is 24/valence= 24/2 = 12

• 1 mEq of magnesium = 12/1000= 0.012 g or 12 mg

• 20 mg/100 ml of magnesium is 200 mg/L

• Therefore, 200 mg divided by 12 = 16.66 mEq/L

Q: Blood work from a cancer patient reveals that the calcium level is five meq/L. How is this expressed in milligrams?

• The atomic weight of calcium = 40

• The equivalent weight of calcium is 40/valence = 40/2 = 20

- 1 mEq of Ca = 20/1000 = 0.020 g or 20 mg

- Therefore 5 mEq = 0..02 x 5 = 0.1 g/L or 100 mg/L

Buffers and Buffering Capacity

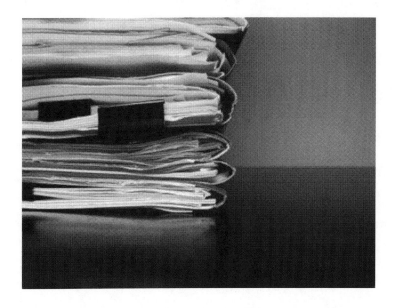

When a small amount of hydrochloric acid is added to water, immediately, there will be an increase in the hydrogen ion concentration. Similarly, when a small amount of sodium hydroxide is added to water, there is a corresponding increase in hydroxyl ions. These biochemical changes occur because water alone does not have the ability to neutralize even the smallest amounts of base or acid. In other words, water has no ability to neutralize the hydrogen or hydroxyl ions or the pH. Similarly, a neutral solution of sodium chloride also is unable to neutralize acids or bases; This means that the final solution is unbuffered.

However, there are some substances or a combination of aqueous solutions that have the ability to maintain the desired pH at a constant level even after the addition of small amounts of a base or an acid; these solutions or chemicals are known as buffers. The ability of these solutions or chemicals to resist changes in pH is known as buffer action, and the solutions are called buffer solutions.

Buffers are often used in pharmacies to maintain and establish ion activity within specific limits. Buffers are commonly used in pharmacies for the following reasons:

• To prepare dosage forms of ophthalmic solutions

• To prepare dosage forms for IV solutions

• To ensure product stability of certain solutions

• Ensure that pharmaceutical assays and tests are functional and not altered by acids or basis

In general, buffer solutions are made of a weak acid and a salt form of the acid, such as sodium acetate and acetic acid, or a weak base and salt of the base, such as ammonium chloride and ammonium hydroxide. Other buffer solutions include disodium phosphate and sodium acid phosphate and boric acid, and disodium borate.

When selecting a buffer system, one must give consideration to the dissociation constant of the weak base of acid to ensure that there is maximum buffering capacity. The dissociation constant reflects the strength of the base or acid; the more readily the acid or base dissociates, the higher the dissociation constant and the stronger the acid.

Drops and Calculations

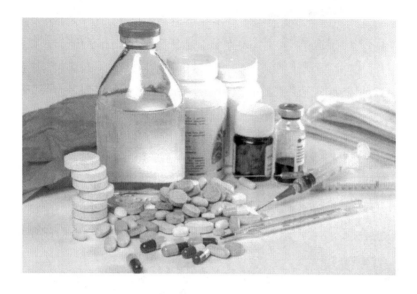

Frequently, drops (abbreviation gtt) are used to measure tiny volumes of liquid medications. Because the drop size can vary immensely with different liquid characteristics, it is not used to represent a specific quantity. However, in order to standardize the use of drops as a measure of volume, the US pharmacopeia has defined the official medicine dropper as being narrow at the delivery end with a round opening with an external diameter of 3 mm.

The dropper should always be held vertically and deliver drops of water that weigh between 45 to 55 mg. The official dropper used in the pharmacy is calibrated so that it can deliver about 20 drops of water per milliliter (i.e., 1 ml of water).

Before a dropper can be used to measure volume, it must be calibrated. Manufacturers of droppers do include a calibrated dropper with prepackaged liquid medications for use by patients. The dropper can be easily calibrated by counting the number of drops of a liquid as it falls into a graduated cylinder until the measurable volume is obtained. The number of drops per unit volume is then recorded, which in most cases is 20 drops/ml.

Frequently the pharmacy technician will need to calculate the dose, Size, number of doses, or the total amount of medication that needs to be dispensed. The equation to be used in all these cases is shown below.

Number of doses - Total quantity/Size of dose

Q: If the pharmacy technician counts 50 drops of a liquid medication to reach the 5 ml mark on a graduated cylinder, how many drops per ml does the dropper deliver?

- 50 drops/X drops = 5 ml/1 ml = 10 drops ml

Q: A patient has been prescribed 250 mg of a drug. How many doses will be contained in a stock of 20 g?

- Number of doses = 20 g (20 x 1000 mg) = 20,000 mg

- Each dose is 250 mg

- Therefore, 20,000/250 = 80 doses

Q: The healthcare provider has prescribed two tablespoons of medication for a 13-year-old. Roughly how many doses will be present in two pints of the stock solution?

- 1 tablespoon = 15 ml.

- Two tablespoon = 30 ml

- 1 pint = 473 ml and hence 2 pints = 946 ml

- Number of doses = 946 ml/30 ml = 31.5 doses

Q: The doctor has written a prescription for a drug that contains 0.040 g of the active ingredient. The stock solution contains 30 g. How many doses of 0.040 g will you be able to make from the stock?

- The total dose is 30 g or 30,000 mg

- The patient's dose is 0.040 g or 40 mg

- Number of doses - 30,000/40 = 750 doses

Q: The pharmacy has 200 ml of elixir that contains 20 doses. How many teaspoonfuls would be prescribed with each dose?

- The size of the dose is 200 ml

- 20 doses means that each dose contains 200 ml/20 = 10 ml

- Each teaspoon is 5 ml, and hence 10 ml will be two teaspoons

Q: The pharmacist has asked you to prepare liquid medication for a patient. The stock solution contains 30 ml contained in 90 doses. The dispensing dropper calibrates 30 drops/ml. How many drops will be prescribed in each dose of the medication?

- The total volume is 30 ml

- Each ml has 30 drops

- Total is 30 x 30 = 900 drops

- Size of the dose = 900 drops divided by 90 doses = ten drops in each dose

Q: A patient has been prescribed a liquid medication that includes two tablespoonfuls three times a day for seven days. How many milliliters of the medication will you provide the patient?

- Number of doses = 3 times daily for 7 days –= 21

- Size of dose = 2 tablespoonfuls or 30 ml

- Total quantity dispensed = 21 x 30 ml =630 ml

Q: A patient has been prescribed a teaspoonful of liquid medication to be taken twice a day for 14 days. How many milliliters of the mixture will you provide the patient?

- Number of doses = two times a day for 14 days = 28 teaspoonfuls

- Total quantity is 28 teaspoonfuls x 5 ml (each teaspoon

is 5 ml) = 140 ml

Q: A 45-year-old diabetic has been prescribed a medication that contains 30 mg. How many grams of the medication will be required to prepare 50 dosage forms?

• Number of doses = 50

• Each dose contains 30 mg

• Total quantity = 50 x 30 mg = 1,500 mg or 1.5 g

Q: A patient with a second-degree burn is prescribed silvadene 2 grams to be applied to his abdomen and chest twice a day for ten days. What is the total number of grams you would dispense?

• Dose frequency is twice a day x ten days = 20 doses total

• The dose per day is 2 g

• Thus, total dose dispensed is 2 g x 20 doses = 40 g

Q: You have been asked by the pharmacist to prepare 100 tablets from a stock of 0.075 g. How many micrograms will each tablet contain?

- First, convert 0.075 g into milligrams = 75 mg

- Then convert this to micrograms which equals 7,500 micrograms

- Total number of tablets is 100 that contain 7,500 micrograms

- Hence each tablet contains 7,500/100 = 75 micrograms

Q: A cough solution contains 8 g of a drug in 250 ml. How many grams will be contained in each tablespoon dose?

- Each tablespoon dose is 15 ml

- Convert 8 g to milligrams = 8,000 mg

- 8,000 mg in 250 ml means that in every ml, there are 8,000/250 ml =32 mg/ml

- Each tablespoon contains 15 ml, and hence the total milligram in each tablespoon is 32 mg x 15 ml = 480 mg or 0.48 g

Q: An analgesic formula contains 80 mg of morphine in 8 fluid ounces. How many milligrams of morphine will be in one teaspoonful dose?

- One fluid ounce = 6 teaspoons

- Eight fluid ounces will contain 48 teaspoons

- There are 80 mg in 48 teaspoons

- Hence one teaspoon will contain 80/48= 1.67 mg

Q: You have been asked to make a 150 ml solution with each teaspoonful containing 3 mg of the drug. How many grams will you require in total?

- One teaspoon = 5 ml; Total volume is 150 ml

- Hence 5 ml/150 ml =3 mg/x; Therefore, x = 90 mg or 0.090 g

Q: The healthcare provider has ordered 250 mg capsules of amoxicillin to be taken twice a day for seven days. How many grams of amoxicillin in total will you dispense?

- Dose duration is seven days, twice a day = 14 doses, Each capsule is 250 mg

- Total dose is 14 doses x 250 mg = 3,500 mg or 3.5 g

Low-Dose and High-Dose Therapies

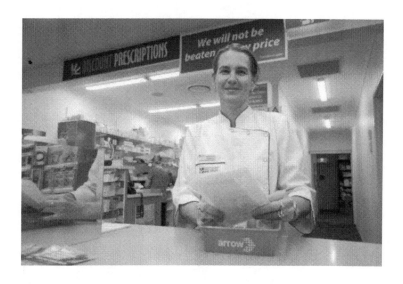

In pharmacy practice, one will encounter both low and high-dose therapies. These therapies are either much smaller or bigger than the standard therapies for some disorders.

The high and low-dose therapies are much different from the normal variation that occurs in patients with advanced age, kidney or liver disease, or low body weight. The classic example of low-dose therapy is the use of aspirin (81mg) instead of the usual 325 mg to reduce the risk of a stroke and heart attack. Another example of low-dose therapy is when menopausal women are prescribed hormonal therapy. The doses prescribed are usually 50% less than the standard doses of the hormones.

High-dose therapy is commonly undertaken in patients with cancer. Chemotherapeutic drugs are given in high doses with the intent to kill cancer cells. Another example where high-dose therapy is used is in the treatment of endometriosis with high-dose progestin.

Another related area where high-dose therapy can occur is in patients who take multiple medications (both non-prescription and prescription) that contain a common ingredient. A classic example is acetaminophen which is present in many other medications. Thus, when calculating drug doses, one must always be aware of similar active ingredients that may also be present in several other drugs.

Pharmacists and pharmacy technicians need to be cognizant that both high-dose and low-dose therapies are frequently used in select patients; the key is to remain vigilant and protect patients against unintended high doses of drugs that can lead to a drug overdose.

Q: A 51-year-old post-menopausal female was taking

0.625 mg of conjugated estrogen until recently. Today, her physician changed to a low-dose formula that contains 0.35 mg conjugated estrogen. How many milligrams less of the conjugated estrogen is the patient taking per week?

- First 0.625 mg minus 0.35 mg = 0.275 mg

- Duration is one week or seven days

- Hence patient is now taking 0.275 mg x 7 days = 1.925 mg

Q: A patient with sarcoidosis has been on high-dose prednisone of 600 mg per day for ten days. The patient's dose has now been decreased to 60 mg/day for the next two months. How much higher was the initial dose compared to the new dose?

- The initial high dose was 600 mg

- Regular dose now is 60 mg

- Therefore, the patient was receiving 600/60 or ten times the regular dose of prednisone

Splitting Tablets

1. Tablets can be split up. A number of medications have a groove or are scored in the middle, which permits one to break them into two equal pieces.

2. This allows flexibility in dosing, especially when the patient is started on half the dose and then gradually titrated to the full dose.

3. Splitting also permits the patient to consume a medication at a strength that may otherwise not be available.

4. Some individuals use tablet splitting to cut both unscored and scored tablets for financial reasons. By splitting the medication, the patient can double his or her supply of the medication.

Unfortunately, splitting a tablet more often than not results in unequal portions of the tablet, and thus the patient receives uneven doses. Furthermore, patients may not be aware that many solid dosage forms should never be crushed, broken, or split but remain intact for adequate drug absorption.

Despite the negatives, tablet splitting is common and often employed in practice for institutional or hospitalized patients who are not able to swallow large solid tablets.

Q: A patient who is unable to afford his blood pressure medications has started to split his 30 mg unscored tablets. However, this has resulted in uneven half tables differing in drug content by 1.75 mg. Assuming a whole tablet is uniform in drug content, calculate the amount of drug in each half of the tablet.

- L = Large, S small

- L + S = 30 mg

- The evenly split tablet is 15 mg

- L - S = 1.75 mg difference

- Therefore, splitting can result in a large tablet that contains L = 15 + 1.75 mg = 16.75 mg

- The smaller tablet will contain 15 - 1.75 mg = 13.25 mg

Standard Units of Activity for Biologicals

1. The potencies of many endocrine products, some antibiotics, vaccines, vitamins, and biological drugs, are

often expressed in terms of their units of activity or in micrograms per milligram.

2. These measures of potency have been approved by the US Food and Drug Administration and set forth in the United States Pharmacopeia (USP). In general, they also conform to international standards defined by the World Health Organization and termed International Units (IU).

3. The degree of activity of a product is often determined by comparing it to a suitable standard, which is usually a USP reference standard. However, there are small variances in potency. For example, the USP monograph on sterile penicillin G mentions that Penicillin G may have a potency between 1,500 to 1,750 units per milligram. The potency or activity of an antibiotic is usually determined by its inhibitory effect on microorganisms.

In most cases, there is a real relationship between the product's unit of activity and measurable quantity (units per milliliter, units per milligram). This relationship can be used as a proportion and/or ratio to determine either the volume or weight or the number of units of activity. The formula is:

Units of activity (given)/ Weight or volume (given) = Units of activity (given or desired)/ Weight or volume (given or desired) units

The most common product whose activity is based on units is insulin. Even though there are many commercially available insulin products depending on their duration of action, time to peak and onset of action, each commercially available insulin is now standardized to contain either 100 insulin units (100-U) or 500 insulin units (500-U) per milliliter of a solution or suspension.

The strength of these insulin products is designated as U-100 and U-500. And as mentioned earlier, dispensing errors can occur when the provider uses an abbreviation like U instead of writing units. A carelessly transcribed 'U' can easily be mistaken for a zero; for example, 200 U could be mistaken for 2,000 units. Thus, it is highly recommended that the word unit be spelled out each and every time. Further, to prevent medication errors, there are special insulin syringes for measuring insulin units; the required dosage is measured in milliliters or units, depending on how the syringe has been calibrated.

Similarly, many biological agents, including toxoids,

vaccines, and immunological serum, may be expressed as units of antigen per milliliter or micrograms.

The potency of a vaccine towards a virus is often expressed in terms of the tissue culture infectious dose (TCID50), meaning the quantity or number of virus particles that can infect 50% of inoculated cultures. Vaccines against viruses may be expressed as units or micrograms of antigen.

The potency of a toxoid is often expressed as flocculating units (LF units). In coordination with several professional organizations, the American Pharmacists Association (APhA) has now included the administration of vaccines as part of professional activities of pharmacists. Hence, Colleges of pharmacy and state pharmacy organizations have created immunization training programs for pharmacists and pharmacy technicians. Depending on the state, pharmacists can administer vaccines to people of all ages as long as they follow established protocols and guidelines.

Units of Activity Calculations

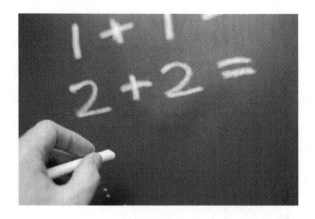

Q: A diabetic patient has been prescribed 30 units of insulin. The stock contains U-100 insulin. How many milliliters of the stock will you use?

- U-100 contains 100 units/ml

- Hence every 10 units equal 0.1 ml

- Therefore, 30 units will be 0.3 ml

Q: A patient with diabetic ketoacidosis is being treated in the emergency room. The physician has prescribed 200 units of insulin to be added to 250 ml of D5W. How many milliliters of the U-500 insulin concentrate will you use?

- U -500 insulin contains 500 units/ml

- Thus, every 0.1 ml contains 50 units

- Therefore 200 units = 0.4 ml

Q: A patient has been ordered 5,000 units of heparin sodium to be added to the dextrose solution for IV infusion. The stock contains 200,000 units in 20 ml. How many milliliters will you use up from the stock?

- Stock = 200,000 units n 20 ml

- Hence each ml = 10,000 units

- To make up 5,000 units, you will withdraw 0.5 ml

Q: An 8-year-old child requires a rabies toxoid following a bite by an unknown dog. The doctor has ordered the patient to receive 20 Lf units. The stock contains 50 Lf units in 5 ml. How many milliliters of the stock will you use?

- Stock is 50 Lf units in 5 ml

- Hence each ml contains 10 Lf units

• If the patient requires 20 Lf units, then this is 2 ml

Q: The rubella virus vaccine live is commercially prepared to contain 5,000 TCID 50 per 0.5 ml. What will be the TCID50 content for a 25 ml multiple dose vials of the vaccine?

• 0.5 ml contains 5,000 TCID 50

• 1 ml will contain 10,000 TCID 50

• Thus 25 ml will contain 25 x 10,000 TCD = 250,000 TCID 50 units

First Quiz

1. In general, what is the drug dose for neonates?

A. 10 micrograms/kg/day

B. 10 mg/kg/day

C. 1 mg/kg/day

D. 100 mg/kg/day

Answer B

At present, the recommended dose for neonates is 10 mg/kg/ day. On the other hand, the adult dose in a 70 kg adult is 150 mg or roughly 2 mg/kg/day.

2. The neonatal period is defined as?

A. First 24 hours of birth

B. First week of life

C. From birth to 1 month of age

D. From birth to 1 year of life

Answer C

1. The neonatal period is from birth to the first month of age.

2. Infancy is defined as a period starting from the first month of birth to the end of the first year of life.

3. Early childhood is the period between the first and the fifth year of life

4. Late childhood is the period between 6-12 years

3. You have been asked to compound a prescription. The directions use the abbreviation 'ppm.' What does ppm stand for?

A. Parts per million

B. Pounds per million

C. Parts per milliliter

D. Parts per milligram

Answer A

PPM is an abbreviation for part per million. It is frequently used to express concentrations of dilute solutions.

4. You have been told that the dose of Nitroglycerin is 0.3 mg. How many doses are contained in 30 mg of the stock?

A. 30

B. 60

C. 100

D. 300

Answer C

1. 30 mg/0.3 mg per dose = 100 doses.

2. In general, when you have a stock supply, you obtain the number of doses by dividing it by the unit dose.

5. You have been asked to calculate the loading dose of an antibiotic. To determine the loading dose, you first need to know:

A. Volume of distribution

B. Rate of excretion

C. Rate of absorption

D. Lipid solubility of the drug

Answer A

1. The loading dose is calculated by the following formula: Loading dose = volume of distribution x desired plasma concentration.

2. The volume of distribution reflects the apparent volume into which the drug is distributed.

3. It is easily calculated by taking the amount of drug at a

specified time and dividing it by the concentration in plasma.

6. How many grains are in 10 grams?

A. 154

B. 15.4

C. 1,540

D. 1.54

Answer: A

1. A gram contains 15.4 grains.

2. Thus, 10 grams will contain 154 grains (ten x 15.4).

7. What is the weight of 100 ml of an alkaline solution whose density is 1.15 g/ml?

A. 100 g

B. 115 g

C. 15 g

D. 203 g

Answer B

1. Weight = density x volume or D = W/V.

2. Weight = 1.15 g/mL x 100 mL = 115 grams.

8. A healthcare provider has written a prescription for 75 mEq of potassium chloride. How many grams will be required?

A. 0.89 g

B. 1.76 g

C. 2.54 g

D. 5.59 g

Answer D

1. To convert milligrams to milliequivalents or vice versa, the below formula can be used: mEq = (mg x valence) / atomic or molecular weight.

2. 75 mEq x 74.6g/1000 mEq = 5.595 g

9. A recently admitted patient has been ordered an IV to run at 100 ml/hr. How long will 1.5 liters last?

A. 10 hours

B. 15 hours

C. 20 hours

D. 30 hours

Answer B

1. The patient is receiving 100 ml/hour, and the total amount of fluid available is 1500 ml.

2. Hence 1,500 ml divided by 100 ml/hr = 15 hours.

10. The student has mixed 750 mg of an antibiotic in 100 ml of normal saline. What is the final concentration?

A. 7.5%

B. 0.75%

C. 7%

D. 0.0785%

Answer: B

750 mg is equal to 0.75 grams, which, when dissolved in 100 ml, is 0.75%.

11. In the cupboard, there is a total of 360 mg of a medication. You are asked to make up 30 mg tablets. How many pills will you make from the stock?

A. 6

B. 8

C. 10

D. 12

Answer D

If there is a total of 360 mg and you need to make up 30 mg tablets, then simply divide 360 by 30= 12

12. The healthcare provider has ordered 30 mg of a medication to be given every 6 hours. How many pills will be needed for seven days?

A. 28

B. 36

C. 68

D. 90

Answer: A

1. If a drug is given every 6 hours, then this equals four tablets a day.

2. In 7 days, this is seven days x 4 pills = 28 pills total.

13. The healthcare provider has written a script for the patient to be dispensed 10 mg of morphine. The pharmacist tells you that the vial contains 50 mg/ml. How much volume should you aspirate in the syringe?

A. 0.4 ml

B. 0.2 ml

C. 0.1 ml

D. 1 ml

Answer B

1. Each ml contains 50 mg of morphine, and you have been asked to dispense 10 mg of morphine.

2. Since each ml contains 50 mg, you will withdraw 0.2 ml (10/50 x 1).

14. A 67-year-old has been admitted with a blood clot in the leg. You send a vial containing 10,000 units of heparin

in 10 ml to the nurse. The doctor has ordered 5,000 units of heparin to be administered as a bolus. How much volume will the nurse draw up in the syringe?

A. 5 ml

B. 10 ml

C. 15 ml

D. 20 ml

Answer: A

1. 10 mL of heparin contains 10,000 units of heparin; therefore, 1 ml contains 1,000 units

2. So if the patient requires 5,000 units of heparin, the nurse will draw up 5 ml

15. A patient is prescribed 200 mL of an antibiotic every 2 hours. How many mL will be delivered in each minute?

A. 1.0 ml

B. 1.7 ml

C. 2 ml

D. 2.4 ml

Answer B

1. The order states 200 ml of the antibiotic every 2 hours. This means the patient receives 100 ml every hour

2. If there are 100 mL per hour, then divide by 60 (number of minutes in one hour); this will give the rate per minute.

3. 100/60 = 1.66, which is rounded off to 1.7 mL per min.

16. How many grams are there in 2.8 kilograms?

A. 28

B. 280

C. 2,800

D. 28,000

Answer C

Each kilogram contains 1,000 grams, so 2.8 kilograms will contain 2,800 grams.

17. A 7-year-old child is prescribed an antibiotic made up of 200 mg/5 ml. The antibiotic is to be taken twice a day for five days. What is the total dose that the child will get in 5 days?

A. 200 mg

B. 400 mg

C. 1,000 mg

D. 2,000 mg

Answer D

1. The dose is 200 mg/5 ml, to be taken twice a day. This equals 400 mg/day.

2. Over five days, the total dose will be 400 mg x 5 days = 2,000 mg.

18. A child is prescribed an antibiotic with a concentration of 200 mg/5 ml. The antibiotic is to be taken twice a day for five days. What is the total volume of the drug that should be dispensed for five days?

A. 5

B. 10

C. 25

D. 50

Answer D

Each day, the child will receive 10 ml, and hence in 5 days, the volume will be 50 mL.

19. While working in a hospital, you see an order by the doctor which states that the patient will receive 1 liter of

normal saline over 10 hours. What will be the flow rate of the drug in ml/hr?

A. 25 mL/hour

B. 50 mL/hour

C. 100 mL/hour

D. 125 mL/hour

Answer C

1. The patient is getting 1,000 mL of fluid over 10 hours. This equals 100 ml/hour.

2. You divide 1,000 ml by 10 hours.

20. A 75-year-old with liver disease has been ordered normal saline intravenously to be administered at a rate of 0.5 ml per minute. What is the total volume of fluid he will receive in 12 hours?

A. 78

B. 160

C. 275

D. 432

Answer D

1. The patient is receiving fluid at a rate of 0.5 ml/min.

2. Multiply by 60 minutes, and this equals 0.6 x 60= 36 ml per hour.

3. Over 12 hours, he will receive 36 ml x 12 hours =432 ml.

21. A 73-year-old with heart failure has been ordered to receive 0.75 liters of normal saline for over 10 hours. What is the calculated flow rate in ml/hr?

A. 25

B. 50

C. 75

D. 100

Answer C

1. The patient is receiving a total of 750 ml (0.75 liters) over 10 hours.

2. This is equal to 750 ml/10 hours, which is 75 ml/hour.

22. The stock solution contains 40% of a substance in 10 ml. A 4% concentration of the substance is needed. What amount of water is needed to make it to 100 mL of a 4% solution?

A. 90

B. 100

C. 110

D. 120

Answer: A

1. Each ml of the original solution is 40%, so to make it

4%, dilute it ten times.

2. Since there is already 10 ml, add 90 mL of water.

23. A patient has been ordered 2,000 ml of normal intravenous saline to be administered over 24 hours. What is the volume he will be administered every hour?

A. 50 ml

B. 75 mL

C. 83 mL

D. 100 mL

Answer C

1. The total volume the patient will get is 2,000 ml over 24 hours.

2. So, during each hour, he will get 83.3 ml (2,000 divided by 24).

24. A patient with Crohn's disease has been prescribed 3 liters of total parenteral nutrition (TPN) at a rate of 125 mL per hour. What will be the total time of infusion?

A. 12 hours

B. 15 hours

C. 20 hours

D. 24 hours

Answer D

1. The total volume of TPN the patient will receive is 3,000 ml.

2. The rate of infusion will be 125 ml/hour.

3. Thus, the duration of the infusion is calculated by dividing 3,000 ml by 125 ml /hr - this equals 24 hour.

25. For children between ages 2-17, which mathematical rule is used to calculate the dosage of medications?

A. Newton

B. Chancy

C. Clark

D. Chaucer

Answer C

1. Clark's rule is a mathematical formula used to calculate dosage in children ages 2-17.

2. The rule is 'weight divided by 150 lbs.) x adult dose = pediatric dosage.'

26. Which of the following reflects Clark's rule to calculate the dose of medications in children?

A. (Height divided by 150 pounds) x adult dose

B. (Weight divided by 150 pounds) x adult dose

C. (Age divided by 150 pounds) x adult dose

D. (Body mass index divided by 150 pounds) x adult dose

Answer B

1. Clark's rule is a formula to calculate drug doses in children. It takes into account the patient weight in pounds divided by the average standard weight of 150 pounds (68 kg). The number obtained is then multiplied by the adult dose of a drug. The final number equals the dose in a child.

2. (Weight divided by 150 lbs.) x adult dose = pediatric dosage.

27. Based on Clark's rule, if an adult is prescribed 250 mg of an antibiotic, how many milligrams will an infant weighing 60 pounds need?

A. 250

B. 100

C. 500

D. 75

Answer B

Using Clark's rule, divide the infant's body weight by 150 and then multiply by 250 mg- this equals 100 mg.

28. You have been asked to calculate the body mass index of a patient. Which of the following formulas will you use?

A. Kg/m^2

B. Kg^2/m^2

C. Kg^2/m

D. Kg/m

Answer A

1. The Body Mass Index (BMI) is a formula that uses the individual's height and weight.

2. The formula for the BMI is kg/m^2, where the individual's weight is in kilograms, and the height is in

meters squared.

3. An individual with a BMI of 25 is considered to be overweight

4. The BMI in healthy people varies from 18.5 to 24.9.

29. What is Fried's rule for calculating the dose of medications in children?

A. Child's age in years/150 x adult dose

B. Child's weight/150 x adult dose

C. Child's age in months/150 x adult dose

D. Child's age in weeks/150 x adult dose

Answer C

1. Fried's rule is a method used to estimate the dose of medication in a child

2. It involves dividing the age of the child in months by 150 and then multiplying the result by the adult dose.

30. When calculating the dose of medications in children, which of the following parameters is not required?

A. Weight

B. Height

C. Age

D. Gender

Answer D

1. There are many methods of calculating doses in children.

2. One usually requires age, weight, height, and body surface area.

3. The child's gender is not required for the dose calculation.

31. A 14-year-old male weighing 98 pounds is prescribed

an antibiotic with a dose of 5 mg/kg. How much drug will he receive?

A. 114

B. 135

C. 222

D. 454

Answer C

1. First, convert the 98 pounds into kilograms. 98 pounds is 44.5 kilograms

2. Then multiply 44.5 kilograms x 5 mg/kg = 222 mg.

32. To convert Fahrenheit to Centigrade, which formula will you use?

A. F= C − (9/5) + 32

B. F= C x (9/5) - 32

C. F= C x (9/5) + 32

D. F= C + (9/5) – 32

Answer C

1. Fahrenheit is a temperature scale where the freezing point of water is at 32 degrees F and the boiling point is 212 degrees.

2. The centigrade scale is where 0 degrees C is the freezing point of water and 100 degrees C is the boiling point of water.

3. Most nations use the centigrade scale for temperature measurements.

4. The formula F= C x (9/5) + 32 is correct.

33. The roman numeral 'L' defines what Arabic number?

A. 5

B. 10

C. 50

D. 100

Answer C

L stands for 50.

34. You have been sent a note by the pharmacist who has written in roman numerals that you should prepare 'CX' number of pills. How many pills will you prepare?

A. 15

B. 40

C. 90

D. 110

Answer D

CX = C + X

C stands for 100, and X stands for 10.

$100 + 10 = 110.$

35. Which of the following correctly identifies room temperature?

A. 73-78 F

B. 72-77 C

C. 68-70 C

D. 90-100 F

Answer: A

Room temperature depends on the season but, in general, varies from 73-78 F or 23-25.5 C.

36. A child weighing 15 kilograms is seen in the Pediatric emergency unit. The healthcare provider has written an order of 5 mg/kg to be administered IV over 4 hours. The total dose the child will receive is?

A. 15 mg

B. 30 mg

C. 50 mg

D. 75 mg

Answer D

The dose is 5 mg per kg, so if the child weighs 15 kilos, then the dose is 5 x 15 = 75 mg.

37. One kilogram is equal to how many pounds?

A. 1.6

B. 1.8

C. 2.2

D. 2.4

Answer C

1. Each kilo is about 2.2 pounds.

2. This number is important to know when converting body weight into body mass index.

38. A 33-year-old female has just purchased 50 antimalarial pills for her trip to Africa. The total cost of the medications was $140. How much does each pill cost?

A. $2.80

B. $3.50

C. $4.00

D. $5.60

Answer A

1. To calculate the cost of the pill, just divide the total cost by the number of pills.

2. This means 140 divided by 50, which is $2.80.

39. The number 19.97 is closest to which of the following integers?

A. 10

B. 98

C. 20

D. 18

Answer C

1. Rounding off numbers is critical.

2. 19.97 is close to twenty

40. Each gram contains how many micrograms?

A. 10

B. 1,000

C. 10,000

D. 1,000,000

Answer D

1. Each gram contains 1000 mg

2. Each mg contains 1,000 micrograms

3. Thus, there are 1,000,000 micrograms in 1 gram.

41. A 100 ml antiseptic solution costs $50. How much will it cost to purchase 20 ml?

A. 8

B. 10

C. 12

D. 16

Answer B

1. 100 ml costs $50; hence every 10 ml costs $5 (50/100 x 10).

2. For 20 mL, the cost is $10.

42. The prescription states that the patient should be dispensed two milliliters of the eye drop. This is the same as which of the following?

A. 2 mL

B. 2 drops

C. 2 mg

D. 2 teaspoons

Answer A

Two milliliters is the same as 2 mL.

43. An antibiotic solution contains 5 mg per ml. This is the same as which of the following?

A. 50 mg per 10 ml

B. 5 mg per 5 ml

C. 5 mg per 1 ml

D. 500 ml per 1 mg

Answer A

5 mg/ml is the same as 50 mg per 10 ml.

44. The healthcare provider has ordered 300 mg of a drug to be administered as a bolus. The original stock is available as 15 mg/ml. How many milliliters should be injected?

A. 5 ml

B. 10 ml

C. 15 ml

D. 20 ml

Answer D

1. The stock contains 15 mg/ml.

2. Thus, to calculate the final volume, divide 300 mg by 15 ml.

3. This equals 20 ml.

45. A patient in the emergency room requires 5 mg of haloperidol stat. The stock solution is labeled as 20 mg/2 ml. To administer 5 mg, how much volume should you aspirate from the stock solution?

A. 0.5 ml

B. 1 ml

C. 1.5 ml

D. 2.0ml

Answer A

1. The stock contains 20 mg in 2 ml or 10 mg in 1 ml or 5 mg in 0.5 ml.

2. Thus, you should draw up 0.5 ml in the syringe

46. The healthcare provider has ordered 20 tablets of a medication that make up a total of 400 mg. How many tablets would you need to make 180 mg of the drug?

A. 2

B. 6

C. 9

D. 12

Answer C

1. 20 tablets make up 400 mg, or in simple items, one tablet makes 20 mg

2. Thus, if you want to make a total of 180 mg, you would need nine tablets (180 divided by 20)

47. The healthcare provider has ordered a patient to

receive 0.35 mg of a drug intravenously. The nurse accidentally administered 3.5 mg. The patient was overdosed by what factor?

A. 1

B. 5

C. 10

D. 20

Answer C

1. The original intended dose was 0.35 mg.

2. The patient received 3.5 mg.

3. This means the patient got ten times the therapeutic dose.

48. The healthcare provider ordered 50 mg of a drug to be administered to the patient intravenously in 10 ml saline. The nurse administered 15 ml of the drug. How much extra drug did the patient receive?

A. 10

B. 25

C. 75

D. 100

Answer B

1. There is 50mg in 10 ml- this equals 5 mg in 1 ml.

2. Thus, if the patient received 15 ml, the 5 mg x 15 ml = 75 mg of the drug.

3. The patient, therefore, received an extra 25 mg (75 mg - 50 mg).

49. On the pharmacy shelf, you have a vial that contains a 1% solution of a local anesthetic. This means that the solution contains:

A. 1 microgram

B. 1 milligram

C. 1 gram

D. 1 kilogram

Answer C

In general, 1% of a solution contains 1 gram of the drug.

50. A gram of dextrose provides 3.4 kcal of energy. How many kcal will be provided by 250 mL of D5W?

A. 21.25 kcal

B. 12.5 kcal

C. 42.5 kcal

D. 17.0 kcal

Answer: C

1. A 5% solution means there are 5 grams of diluent (dextrose in this case) per 100 mL.

2. Determine the number of grams of dextrose in 250 mL

of D5W.

3. Set up a ratio: 5 g/100 mL - Xg/250 mL; X - 12.5 g.

4. Therefore: 12.5 g x 3.4 kcal/g = 42.5 kcal.

Second Quiz

1. A 33-year-old with diabetic ketoacidosis is admitted with significant hypokalemia. The physician has ordered a 3% KCL solution for infusion in 400 mL of saline. How much total potassium will be infused in the patient?

A. 3 grams

B. 12 grams

C. 8 grams

D. 15 grams

Answer B

1. One percent solution contains 1 gram in 100 ml

2. A 3% solution of KCL contains 3 grams of potassium.

3. Therefore, 400 mL will have 4 x 3 = 12 grams.

2. How much water should be added to 1,000 ml of 60%

alcohol to prepare a 30% solution?

A. 200 mL

B. 1,000 mL

C. 750 mL

D. 500 mL

Answer B

1. Initial solution (IS) = 60%, Initial volume = 1,000 mL,

2. Final solution (FS) = 30%, and Final volume (FV) = unknown.

3. (60%)(1,000 mL) = (30%)(FV), where FV = 2,000 mL.

4. FV - IV = 2000-1,000= 1,000 mL.

3. You have a stock solution of an antibiotic at 10 mg/ml. How much volume will you require to make 40 ml of 0.5 mg/ml solution?

A. 2 ml

B. 5 ml

C. 7 ml

D. 10 ml

Answer A

1. Initial solution is 10 mg/ml. The final volume is unknown.

2. Final solution is 0.5 mg/ml, and the final volume is 40 ml

3. (10 mg/ml)(IV) - (0,5 mg)(40ml)= 2 ml

4. You have been asked to make a 50 ml dilution of drug A with a concentration of 100 mcg/ml from a stock solution of 1 mg/ml. How much of the diluent will you need?

A. 25 mL

B. 35 mL

C. 45 mL

D. 50 mL

Answer C

1. (IS)(IV) = (FS)(FV)

2. IS = 1 mg/mL = 1,000 mcg/mL, IV is unknown,

3. FS = 100 mcg/mL and FV = 50 mL.

4. (1,000 mcg/mL)(IV) = (100 mcg/mL)(50 mL), IV = 5 mL.

5. The amount of diluent = (FV - IV) = 50 mL - 5 mL = 45 mL.

5. You have been asked to prepare 40 ml of a 1:5 solution of drug Y. In stock, you have a 40% solution. How many milliliters of the stock solution will you use?

A. 20 ml

B. 22ml

C. 25 ml

D. 30 ml

Answer A

1. First, convert the ratio (1:5) to a percentage that equals 20%

2. Formula is (IS)(IV) =(FS)(FV)

3. IS is 40%, and IV is unknown. FS is 20% and FV is 40 ml

4. (40%)(IV)= (20%) (40ml)= 20 ml

6. If a patient receives Ringers lactate at a rate of 75 ml/hr for 24 hours, what will be the total volume of fluid administered?

A. 1,000 ml

B. 1,400 ml

C. 1,800 ml

D. 2,000 ml

Answer C

1. Patient receives RL at 75 ml per hour

2. In 24 hours, he will receive 75 ml x 24 hours =1,800 ml

7. A patient has been prescribed a total volume of 2,400 ml of normal saline over 20 hours. What will be the flow rate per hour?

A. 100 ml/hr

B. 120 ml/hr

C. 140 ml/hr

D. 150 ml/hr

Answer B

Rate = Volume/Time (hour) = 2,400 mL/20 hour = 120 mL/hour.

8. The hospital pharmacy receives an order to make up 500 mg of a drug in 250 ml of normal saline. The doctor has stated that the infusion time is 3 hours. How many ml per hour will the patient receive?

A. 50 ml/hr

B. 83.3 ml/hr

C. 75 ml/hr

D. 90.4 ml/hr

Answer B

1. Total volume is 250 ml

2. Duration of IV infusion is 3 hours

3. Hence each hour patient will get 250 ml/3 hr = 83.3 ml/hr

9. The cardiac surgeon has ordered a heparin dose of 150

units/kg for a patient weighing 220 pounds. The stock solution contains 10,000 units of heparin/ml. How many ml will you prepare?

A. 0.5 ml

B. 1.0 ml

C. 1.5 ml

D. 2.0 ml

Answer C

1. First, convert 220 pounds to kilograms; 220/2,2 = 100 kilos

2. The patient needs 150 units per kg, so the total dose will be 150 units x 100 kilos= 15,000 units of heparin

3. Each vial contains 10,000 units of heparin per ml. so you will need 1.5 ml

10. You have been asked to calculate the pharmacy's overhead for the year 2022. The salary of the pharmacist

is $80,000, the pharmacy technician's salary is $35,000, Pharmaceutical drugs $4 million, Licenses $5,000, rent $120,000, Insurance $4,500, Utilities $4000, supplies $75,000, and software $100,000. The overhead is:

A. $4 423 500

B. $4 400 500

C. $4 300 550

D. $4 350,400

Answer A

1. Overhead is the sum of all the expenses.

2. $80,000 + $35,000 + $4, 000 000 + $5,000 +$120,000. + 4,500 + $4,0000 + $75,000 + $100, 000= $4,423 500

11. You have a 1:2 stock solution of a drug X. You have been asked to prepare 50 ml of drug X with a 1:4 solution. How many milliliters of the 1:2 solution will you use?

A. 22 mL

B. 43 mL

C. 50 mL

D. 100 mL

Answer B

1. This is a dilution calculation that is best done using ratios.

2. In stock = 1:2

3. Initial volume (IV) = unknown

4. Final solution = 1:4

5. Final volume = 50 mL.

6. (1:2)(IV) = (1:4)(50 mL) = 43 mL = IV.

12. In your pharmacy, the glucometer has an Average Wholesale Price of $50. It retails for $90 and has a dispensing cost of $5. What is the gross profit made by the pharmacy?

A. $10

B. $20

C. $35

D. $40

Answer D

1. Gross profit is calculated by subtracting the Average Wholesale Price from the retail price.

2. Thus, $90 minus $50= $40

13. Your pharmacy is selling a medication that costs $12 with a dispensing fee of $4 for $20. What is the markup of the drug?

A. $4

B. $8

C. $10

D. $12

Answer B

1. The markup price is equal to the retail price of the drug ($20) minus the drug costs.

2. Cost is $12; hence the markup is $20-$12, which equals $8

14. Your pharmacy is selling a drug that costs $15 for a retail price of $25. What is the markup rate for this medication?

A. 33%

B. 43%

C. 56%

D. 66%

Answer D

1. Markup dollars divided by the cost times 100 gives the

rate.

2. Calculate the markup: retail price ($25.00) - cost ($15.00) = $10.00.

3. Divide the markup dollars ($10.00) by the cost ($15.00) and multiply by 100: ($10.00/$15.00) x 100 = 66%.

15. A recently approved medication has an Average Acquisition Cost of $90 and a dispensing fee of $20. It retails for $130. What is the net profit made by the pharmacy?

A. $10

B. $20

C. $25

D. $30

Answer B

1. The net profit is the retail price of $130.00 minus the cost of the product, $90, minus expenses of $20.

2. $130 − ($90 + $20) = $20.00.

16. At your pharmacy, the automatic sphygmomanometer costs $100. The overhead for your pharmacy is $5. However, the store wants to make a net profit of $60. What should be the selling price of the device?

A. $145

B. $155

C. $165

D. $175

Answer C

1. First, add the cost of the machine, $100, to the overhead cost, which is $5, to bring the total cost to $105

2. To calculate the selling price; add the total cost and net profit together; hence $105 plus $60 = $165

17. The pharmacy receives a 3% discount if it pays the wholesaler within 30 days. How much will it pay the wholesaler if the invoice for $30,000 is paid within this time period?

A. $900.00

B. $19,100

C. $29,100

D. $39,100

Answer C

1. The pharmacy receives a 3% discount from the total bill if the costs are paid within 30 days.

2. If the invoice is $30,000, then 3% of this is 0.03 x 30,000 = $900

3. Thus, the final bill will be $30,000 minus $900 = $29,100.

18. A child weighing 20 kg has been ordered 10 mg of

medication. The maximum dose is 1 mg /kg. What is the calculated dose of the medication that the child will receive?

A. 0.5 mg/kg

B. 0.7 mg/kg

C. 1.4 mg/kg

D. 2.4 mg/kg

Answer A

1. Calculate the dose on a per-kilogram basis

2. Dose is 10 mg, and the child weighs 20 kg; therefore, the child will receive 0.5 mg/kg, which is less than the maximum safe dose

19. A child weighing 54 pounds has been prescribed an antibiotic with a dose of 250 mg three times a day. The safe dose range in this population is 10-50 mg/kg per day. Which of the following is the correct and safe total daily

dose for the child?

A. 12. 5 mg/kg per day, safe

B. 25 mg/kg per day, unsafe

C. 30.6 mg/kg per day, safe

D. 50.4 mg/kg per day, safe

Answer C

1. First, convert the body weight from pounds to kilos: 54 pounds = 24.5 kilos

2. Divide 250 mg by the body weight of 24.5 kilos to determine the amount in one dose- 250 mg/24.5 = 10.2 mg/kg per dose

3. The child receives the dose three times a day which equals 10.2 mg/kg per dose x 3 = 30.6 mg/kg/day

4. The dose is in the middle of the safety range and considered safe

20. A patient has been prescribed a drug at 20 mg/kg/day in three divided doses. If the patient weighs 50 pounds, how much drug should be prescribed per day?

A. 240 mg

B. 454 mg

C. 500 mg

D. 654 mg

Answer B

1. First convert pounds to kilograms, 50 lbs = 2.2 lbs/ kg = 22.2 kg of body weight.

2. Multiply the daily dose of 20 mg/kg/day times the body weight of 22.2 kg to obtain the correct dose - 20 mg/kg/day X 22.2 kg = 454 mg/day.

21. A 71-year-old weighing 180 pounds is in heart failure. The doctor has ordered dopamine at 200 mg in 500 ml of normal saline at a rate of 5 mcg/kg/min. What will be the

final concentration of the solution in mcg/ml

A. 4 mcg/mL

B. 40 mcg/mL

C. 400 mcg/mL

D. 4,000 mcg/mL

Answer C

1. 200 milligrams dopamine in 500 mL = 0.4 mg/mL.

2. Convert mg to micrograms: 1 mg = 1,000 mcg, 0.4 mg = 400 mcg.

3. The final concentration of dopamine will be 400 mcg/mL.

22. How many grams of a compound (99.9% w/w) must be added to 1 gallon of water to produce a solution containing 0.35% wt./vol of the compound? (hint 1 gallon contains 3,785 ml)

A. 3.25 g

B. 8.5 g

C. 13.2 g

D. 14.5 g

Answer C

1. One gallon contains 3,785 mL.

2. 3,785 mL x 0.35% = 13.2 g.

23. A 55-year-old has been ordered to take an antibiotic containing 4 mg every 6 hours. You have a stock solution that contains 4 mg/ml with a total volume of 50 ml. How many days will the stock last?

A. 4.3 days

B. 7.4 days

C. 8.3 days

D. 10 days

Answer C

1. The content of the vial will be 50 mL X 4 mg/mL = 200 mg.

2. The amount of the drug prescribed = 4 mg x 4 times a day = 24 mg/day.

3. Hence total dose of 200 mg divided by 24 = 8.3 days.

24. A vial contains an antibiotic with a concentration of 1000 units/ml in 10 ml. The healthcare provider has ordered that the patient be administered 6000 units as a single intramuscular dose. How much volume of the drug should be drawn up?

A. 4 mL

B. 2 mL

C. 1 mL

D. 6 mL

Answer D

1. Each vial contains 1,000 units/mL, and 6000 units are needed.

2. Thus, one should divide 6,000/1,000. This equals 6 mL.

25. An antibiotic with a concentration of 1,000,000 units has been dissolved in 5 ml of normal saline. The healthcare provider has ordered the patient to receive 300,000 units. How many mL should be drawn up in a syringe?

A. 0.5 mL

B. 1 mL

C. 1.5 mL

D. 2 mL

Answer C

1. Each vial contains 5 ml with 1,000,000 units; thus, each ml contains 200,000 units.

2. Thus, if you want 300,000 units, you draw up 1.5 mL.

26. The healthcare provider has prescribed an in-patient to receive 70 mg of an antibiotic. The pharmacist sends a 10 ml vial that contains 20 mg/ml. How much volume from the vial should the nurse aspirate?

A. 1.8 ml

B. 2.5 ml

C. 3.5 ml

D. 7 ml

Answer C

1. The provider has ordered 70 mg, and the vial contains 20 mg/ml.

2. To make 70 mg, the nurse needs to draw up 3.5 ml from the vial.

27. The healthcare provider has ordered 12.5 mg of an antibiotic solution. The stock solution contains 50 mg in 2 ml. What volume of the stock solution will you aspirate in the syringe for the patient?

A. 0.5 ml

B. 1.0 ml

C. 1.5 ml

D. 1.75 ml

Answer A

1. The vial contains 50 mg in 2 ml, which makes it 25 mg in 1 ml. or 12.5 mg in 0.5 ml.

2. Thus, to administer 12.5 mg, you will draw up 0.5 ml of the stock solution.

28. You have been asked to add 20 units of regular insulin to the total parenteral nutrition formula. The pharmacist has sent over a vial that contains 50 units of regular

insulin in 5 ml. What volume of the regular insulin will you aspirate from the vial and add to the TPN formula?

A. 1 ml

B. 1.5 ml

C. 2.0 ml

D. 5 ml

Answer C

1. The 50 units of regular insulin are made up of 5 ml. Thus one ml contains ten units. Two ml will contain 20 units

2. Since the TPN solution needs 20 units, draw up 2 ml.

29. You come across a 4% drug solution in 100 ml. How many grams of the drug does the solution contain?

A. 0.40 gram

B. 1 gram

C. 2 grams

D. 4 grams

Answer D

If there is 4% of a drug, this indicates that there are 4 grams in 100 mL.

30. A child weighing 65 pounds needs an antibiotic. The adult dose of the antibiotic is 400 mg. What is the dose for the child based on Clark's rule?

A. 73 mg

B. 173 mg

C. 273 mg

D. 373 mg

Answer B

1. Clark's rule is (patient weight/150) x adult dose

2. Thus, according to Clark's rule, this is (65/150) x 400 = 173 mg.

31. A child has been prescribed 250 mg/5 ml of a drug to be taken twice a day for seven days. What is the total volume of the drug that should be dispensed for seven days?

A. 320

B. 280

C. 140

D. 70

Answer D

Each day, the child will get 10 ml (250mg/5 ml twice a day), and hence in 7 days, the volume will be 70 mL.

32. A 66-year-old patient is to receive 1.1 liters of normal saline over 6 hours. What will be the flow rate in ml/hour?

A. 80

B. 183

C. 125

D. 640

Answer B

1. The patient is getting a total of 1,100 mL over 6 hours.

2. This is equal to 1,100/6- which is 183 ml/hour.

33. A 44-year-old has been ordered 7.5 mg of morphine. The pharmacist sends over a vial containing 25 mg/ml to the nurse's station. How much volume will the nurse draw?

A. 0.1 ml

B. 0.2 ml

C. 0.3 ml

D. 0.5 ml

Answer C

1. Each ml contains 25 mg or 5 mg in every 0.2 ml or 2.5 mg in every 0.1 ml

2. If the nurse wants to administer 7.5 mg, then she needs to draw 0.3 ml.

34. A 66-year-old has just been diagnosed with a thrombus in her left leg and requires heparin. The doctor has ordered an immediate bolus of 5,000 units of heparin. The pharmacist sends a vial containing 10,000 units of heparin in 5 ml to the nurse's station. How much will the nurse draw from the vial?

A. 0. 5 ml

B. 1 ml

C. 1.5 ml

D. 2.5 ml

Answer D

1. There are 10,000 units of heparin in 5 ml; hence each ml will contain 2,000 units.

2. If the patient requires 5,000 units, the nurse will draw 2.5 ml

35. The healthcare provider has written a prescription for 100 mEq of potassium chloride. How many grams will you need to make this weight?

A. 2.45 g

B. 3.84 g

C. 5.77 g

D. 7.46 g

Answer D

1. Molar mass of potassium chloride is 74.6 g/mol.

2. 100 mEq x 74.6 g/1,000 mEq = 7.46. g.

36. You have a 100 ml solution of an acid whose density is 1.20 g/ml. What is the weight of the solution?

A. 30 g

B. 60 g

C. 120 g

D. 240 g

Answer C

1. Density = weight/volume or weight = density x volume.

2. Weight = 1.20 g/mL x 100 mL = 120 grams.

37. Your pharmacy recently bought a case of 2,000 tablets of drug X for $800. The pharmacist has indicated a markup of 150%. What will be the selling price for 50 tablets?

A. 10

B. 50

C. 200

D. 250

Answer B

1. Cost per tablet = $800/2000 = $0.4 per tablet.

2. Markup would be $0.4 X 150%, or $0.60.

3. Cost + Markup = Selling price.

4. $0.40 + $0.60 = $1 per tablet. The selling price for 50 tablets would be $1 X 50 = $50.

38. Your pharmacy has an inventory value of $1,000,000 with pharmacy sales of $4,000,000. What is the inventory turnover rate?

A. 1

B. 2

C. 4

D. 10

Answer C

1. Calculate inventory turn by dividing total sales by the inventory value.

2. Sales 4,000,000/1,000,000 = 4 inventory turns.

39. In the USA, what is the maximum amount of time that can be assigned to a repackaged drug?

A. 1 week

B. 1 month

C. 3 months

D. 6 months

Answer D

The maximum amount of time that can be assigned to a

repackaged medication is six months.

40. Convert 10 grams to grains.

A. 1,540 grains

B. 154 grains

C. 15.4 grains

D. 1.54 grains

Answer: B

1. 15.4 grains = 1 gram.

2. Thus, 10 grams x 15.4 grains/gram = 154 grains.

41. You have been asked to dissolve 750 mg of a medication in 100 ml of sterile water. What will be the final concentration of the solution?

A. 7.5%

B. 0.75%

C. 7%

D. 0.075%

Answer B

750 mg is 0.75 grams, which is 0.75%.

42. A 77-year-old patient is receiving an IV at 90 mL/hour. How long will 2.0 liters last?

A. 11 hours

B. 18 hours

C. 22 hours

D. 30 hours

Answer C

The patient is receiving a total of 2,000 ml, and the rate is 90 mL/hr; this equals 2,000/90 or 22 hours.

43. A 71-year-old with heart failure is receiving normal saline intravenously at a rate of 0.5 mL per minute. What is the total volume of fluid he will receive in 6 hours?

A. 75

B. 155

C. 180

D. 90

Answer C

1. The patient is getting 0.5 mL per minute. Multiply by 60 minutes, and this is 30 ml per hour

2. In 6 hours, he will receive 6 x 30 = 180 ml

44. Convert 1.8 kilograms into micrograms.

A. 1,800

B. 18,000

C. 180,000

D. 1 800,000

Answer D

1. Each kilogram is 1,000 grams, and each gram contains 1,000 micrograms

2. So 1.8 kilo = 1800 mgs or 1,800 x 1,000 = 1,800,000 micrograms

45. You have been given a solution of 10 ml containing 20% of drug A. The pharmacist wants you to make a 2% concentration of drug A. How much water will you add to make it 100 ml of a 2% solution?

A. 90

B. 70

C. 50

D. 120

Answer A

1. Each ml of the original solution is 20%, so to make it 2% dilute it ten times.

2. Since there are already 10 ml, you need to add 90 mL of water.

46. A patient in a nursing home has been prescribed ringer lactate for dehydration. The doctor has ordered a total of 1,500 ml over 24 hours. What will be the rate of infusion?

A. 750 mL

B. 100 mL

C. 62.5 mL

D. 83.3 mL

Answer: C

If the total volume in 24 hours is 1,500 mL, then divide it by 24, and the answer is 62.5 mL per hour.

47. The Arabic equivalent of the Roman numerals XXXIV is?

A. 26

B. 34

C. 44

D. 56

Answer B

X = 10 (x 3 equals 30), plus IV = , so the total is 34.

48. You have a prescription from another pharmacist which has the following roman numerals: '3X.' How many pills will you dispense?

A. 30

B. 13

C. 7

D. 3

Answer C

1. With roman numerals, if the letter of low value is placed before another letter of greater value, then the lower number is subtracted from the higher value.

2. $10 - 3 = 7$

49. A 22-year-old female weighing 102 pounds has been prescribed medication at a dose of 3 mg/kg. What's the total amount of drug she should receive?

A. 49.9 mg

B. 139 mg

C. 75.4 mg

D. 44.4 mg

Answer B

1. First, convert the pounds into kilograms. 102 pounds is 46.3 kilograms.

2. Then multiply 46.3. kilograms X 3 mg/kg. The answer is 139 mg.

50. The pharmacist has purchased a glucose meter for $50 from the wholesaler. He wants to make a profit and hence has marked up the price by 100%. What will be the selling price?

A. $50

B. $100

C. $150

D. $200

Answer: B

1. $50 (cost) + [100% X $50 = $50.00 (markup)] = $50 + $50 = $100 (selling price).

2. Cost + Markup = Selling Price.

Final Thoughts

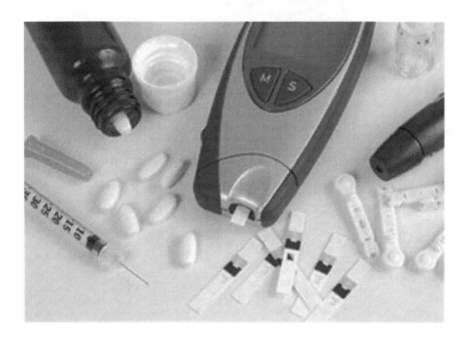

The world of pharmaceuticals is vast and requires skill to navigate. I hope that my book has assisted you on your educational journey.

Would you please do me a favor? If you have not already done so, would you leave a review online wherever you purchased this book? I plan on reading all of the customer reviews so I can make my next book even better. Thank you in advance; I wish you the best of luck!

Made in the USA
Las Vegas, NV
13 January 2024

84317025R00103